"Like a skillful surgeon encouraging us through a difficult but necessary procedure, Curt Thompson works to set us free from our old stories in which shame holds us captive to the common, core fear of having our inadequacies exposed. Naming that fear is the road to healing and hope, not only in our own soul but also in our marriages, families, communities, churches and places of work. This is a challenging but profoundly life-giving book that teaches us—using many fascinating stories from Thompson's work as a psychiatrist—how to relate our inner world of thoughts, emotions and body sensations to the intriguing findings of contemporary brain science, and above all to the biblical story of God's longing that we live openly in the light of his love, delight and grace. Thus new stories are told."

**Richard Winter,** professor of practical theology and director of counseling, Covenant Theological Seminary

"With the discerning eye of a wise therapist, Curt Thompson shows that shame is not just a consequence of human sin but also a toxic 'emotional weapon' that stands at the root of sin, distancing us from God, from others and from our own place in God's beautiful and good creation. But Thompson reminds us that in Christ, God wants to heal our shame. Shame tells us that we are unworthy and unloved and that we should retreat and protect ourselves. But the gospel frees us to be vulnerable and therefore to be rescued from shame, because we are known and loved by the one who assumed our shame that we might enter into his joy. If you experience shame—which is to say, if you are a human being—then this book bears good news for you."

**Warren Kinghorn,** Duke University Medical Center and Duke Divinity School

"This is a psychiatrist's version of *The Screwtape Letters*, exposing the most insidious, destructive tool used against humanity since creation. Never has a book so clearly revealed to me that our struggle is not against flesh and blood. Using his background in interpersonal neurobiology, Dr. Thompson shines a bright light of love on the domains of darkness in the layers of our minds to expose and expel the power of shame. This is a life-changing book."

**Nicole Johnson,** dramatist with Women of Faith, author of *Fresh Brewed Life*

"There may be 'no condemnation for those who are in Christ Jesus,' but many of us don't behave that way. Read this excellent guide for unearthing the things in your own life that are preventing you from being set free."

**Rob Moll,** editor at large, *Christianity Today*, author of *What Your Body Knows About God*

"As a wise man once testified, 'The worst moment in life is when you get everything you ever wanted and discover that it's not enough.' As Curt Thompson so clearly and compassionately demonstrates, it is this insidious not-enough-ness that embodies the very soul of shame. Anyone who longs to break free from the shackles of shame will find a wide array of valuable tools within the pages of this book."

**David Williams,** general superintendent, Evangelical Friends Church

"Though shame often exerts hidden, destructive power over us, *The Soul of Shame* invites us to find freedom with each other and in God's story of love for us. Curt Thompson weaves together experience, insightful stories, science and Scripture to invite us into a story of healing and flourishing together. This excellent book will help to guide my thoughts and relationships for a long time."

**Kent Annan,** author of *After Shock* and *Following Jesus Through the Eye of the Needle*

"In *The Soul of Shame* Curt Thompson deftly combines the emerging field of interpersonal neurobiology with Christian theology, shaped and understood by his own practice as a therapist and his multiple roles as husband, father, son, brother, friend and follower of Jesus. As an educator seeking to serve children living amidst the grim realities of urban poverty, I often discuss our desire to cultivate the ideal conditions for human flourishing and shalom, and Curt Thompson has provided me with the language to name and better understand one of our greatest enemies— shame. But more importantly, *The Soul of Shame* provides a framework for scorning shame and allowing vulnerability, joy and community to thrive."

**Bentley Craft,** head of school, West Dallas Community School

"Through a masterfully woven blend of psychology, neurobiology, theology and real-life stories of patients he's known, Thompson charts a path through the shadowy territory of shame and leads us out the other side to hope and healing. The message here is a dose of good news for all of us who are thirsty for freedom from shame's insistent voice telling us that we are not enough. It turns out that the path to that freedom is paradoxical—as we trust enough in God's love to face the very vulnerability we fear, shame is cut off at the knees. Read this book and discover a story about who you really are that will lead you to increasing freedom and wholeness."

**David A. Schrader,** Full Circle Group

"In *The Soul of Shame*, Dr. Curt Thompson reveals how the repressed origins of fear lead to feelings of vulnerability that direct human behavior, often unconsciously. He illustrates how experiences, often from childhood, are transformed into seeds of shame that shape human behavior for a lifetime, influence decision-making and form the stimulus for unconscious responses in our day-to-day personal and professional lives for decades. This is an important read for many audiences seeking advanced insight into human behavior: individuals on a journey toward self-discovery, parents striving to lay a strong foundation for emotional health and maturity in their children, as well as business leaders seeking to provide the safety needed to achieve breakthrough innovation in the workplace."

**Janey Price Nodeen,** president, Burke Consortium, Inc.

# THE
# SOUL
## OF
# SHAME

## RETELLING THE STORIES WE
## BELIEVE ABOUT OURSELVES

## CURT THOMPSON, MD

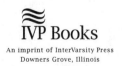
IVP Books
An imprint of InterVarsity Press
Downers Grove, Illinois

*InterVarsity Press*
*P.O. Box 1400, Downers Grove, IL 60515-1426*
*ivpress.com*
*email@ivpress.com*

*InterVarsity Press® is the book-publishing division of InterVarsity Christian Fellowship/USA®, a movement of students and faculty active on campus at hundreds of universities, colleges and schools of nursing in the United States of America, and a member movement of the International Fellowship of Evangelical Students. For information about local and regional activities, visit intervarsity.org.*

*All Scripture quotations, unless otherwise indicated, are taken from THE HOLY BIBLE, NEW INTERNATIONAL VERSION®, NIV® Copyright © 1973, 1978, 1984, 2011 by Biblica, Inc.™ Used by permission. All rights reserved worldwide.*

*While any stories in this book are true, some names and identifying information may have been changed to protect the privacy of individuals.*

*Cover design: Cindy Kiple*
*Interior design: Beth McGill*
*Images: © MrsWilkins/iStockphoto*

*ISBN 978-0-8308-4433-3 (print)*
*ISBN 978-0-8308-9874-9 (digital)*

*Printed in the United States of America* ∞

**Library of Congress Cataloging-in-Publication Data**
*Thompson, Curt, 1962-*
*The soul of shame : retelling the stories we believe about ourselves / Curt Thompson, M.D.*
   *pages cm*
*Includes bibliographical references and index.*
*ISBN 978-0-8308-4433-3 (hardcover : alk. paper)*
*1. Shame—Religious aspects—Christianity. 2. Shame—Biblical teaching. I. Title.*
*BT714.T46 2015*
*233'.5—dc23*

                                                                                              *2015018835*

**P** 24 23 22 21 20 19 18 17 16
**Y** 36 35 34 33 32 31 30 29 28 27 26 25 24 23 22

For David Harper, with deep and lasting affection.

# Contents

# The Story That Shame Is Trying to Tell

This is a book about shame. You might wonder why we need another book about the topic. Shame has made an impressive resurgence in the popular media as well as the academy. It has been the focus of helpful, impressive work by researchers such as Brené Brown and has become a go-to topic of conversation for talk shows. At one level this makes sense, given the place that shame has in our lives. For indeed, it is everywhere, and there is virtually nothing left untainted by it.

From our family at home to the one at church. From the bedroom to the boardroom. From school to work to play. From the art studio to the science and technology lab. It is a primal emotional pigment that colors the images of everything: our bodies, our marriages and our politics; our successes and failures; our friends and enemies, especially the God of the Bible, who may at times feel like both. It starts and (surprisingly) ends wars, only to start them again. It fuels injustice and creates our excuses for doing little if anything about it. It is a featured tool for motivating students, athletes and employees. It enables us to conveniently remain separate from those we disagree with and who make us feel uncomfortable, while keeping to those who will only tell us what we want to hear.

And yet. Given the airplay it has received recently, one would think we would have it all pretty much packaged and wrapped. We simply need to do what we now know we can do to manage the problem. Is it really so complicated that we need yet another angle to approach it from?

And yet. If the healing of shame were so straightforward, why are we still so easily buckled by it? If you're reading this, you may perceive faint awareness of shame's place in your life, but perhaps you are intrigued because more and more people are talking about it. Or maybe you wrestle with shame rather frequently, seeing it or suspecting it in much of your life. Beyond this, you may be tormented by it or even feel wrangled to the ground by it; you would excise it from your life if you could. Its presence and activity are undeniable, as are your seemingly impotent tactics for addressing it.

Despite all we know about shame, containing it, let alone disposing of it, is a bit like grasping for mercury: the more pressure you use to seize it, the more evasive it becomes. In my previous book, *Anatomy of the Soul*, I explored the intersection of Christian spiritual formation and findings from the emerging field of interpersonal neurobiology. As I have had the privilege of walking with people in the context of that work, one theme continues to raise its head. No matter the setting, whether it is a retreat I am leading, a business with which I am consulting, a conference I am addressing or patients I am sitting with, shame eventually makes its way to center stage. Though unpleasant, its interpersonal neurobiological effects are fascinating, while it simultaneously bends and twists our narratives into painful story lines. It is ubiquitous, seeping into every nook and cranny of life. It is pernicious, infesting not just our thoughts but our sensations, images, feelings and, of course, ultimately our behavior. It just doesn't seem to go away.

It is instructive to observe the way we respond to recent research that has so helpfully awakened us to shame's presence and the necessary place of vulnerability in addressing it. Given the tidal wave of interest (as of this writing Brown's TED talks have had over ten million views) one would think that we were discovering shame for the first time in history. Indeed, even in the hallowed halls of psychoanalysis, shame has long remained in the shadows and has only in the last few decades been found important enough for writers and clinicians to bring it into the light.

But then again, haven't we been here before? In 1988 John Bradshaw gave us *Healing the Shame That Binds You* and the PBS series that followed. It has helped literally millions of readers and viewers. You would think, given this resource, that we would have made major gains in correcting our behavior as a culture and nation. But strikingly shame seems to have effectively slinked into the shadows, only now again being ferreted out by a new wave of hunters. Apparently, we either forgot what Bradshaw and others were saying or never paid attention in the first place. It seems that virtually every generation has to go about the process of discovering shame again for the first time. This all reminds us that for all of our hope in cultural progression, in the deepest recesses of our souls, we sense that that is an illusion.

Upon reflection, perhaps this cycle is exactly what we should expect from shame. It likes to do its work and, when exposed, retreat into the shadows, only then to remerge no less potently than before. But it is also possible that the way shame operates is an extension of something larger and more sinister. And to realize this is also to realize that the healing of shame is not merely going to be a function of greater social awareness of it or a novel mental health exercise. To effectively enter into the healing of shame requires us to know the place it holds in our story as a human race, and that requires us to know which story, exactly, we believe we are living in. This book, therefore, is not just a book about shame. It is a book about storytelling—the stories we tell about ourselves (which of course include others and especially God), how we tell them and, more importantly, the story that shame is trying to tell about us.

## OUR STORY AND SHAME'S STORY

Of all the things that set us apart from the rest of creation as humans, one feature stands out: we tell stories. No other creatures we know of tell stories the way we do. (Well, it's possible that certain plants and animals tell stories. They're just not telling *us*.) Whether we know it or not, and whether we intend to or not, we live our lives telling stories; in fact, we don't really know how to function and *not* tell them. We tell them for many reasons. We do so not just to describe what we are doing but to make sense of what we have done. Some may be familiar with the idea of our having a narrator that is infrequently quiet, informing us of the life we are living, and not always using only words. Each of us lives within a story we believe we occupy. Not all of us are equally conscious of this. Depending on which story we believe is the *big* story, the one that unites all the other stories and is the real story about the world, shame will be understood and dealt with accordingly.

In this book I will examine shame in the context of the biblical narrative. And, as I will suggest more directly later, if shame is not understood in this context, it will become a powerful driving force in telling a different story. There are alternatives to the biblical story that consider shame differently than we will in this book. For example, it can be comprehended within some version of a naturalistic evolutionary framework, but for my money that story has very little drama and no purpose. It goes nowhere. It ends with the earth and humanity either flaming out or freezing up, and we are left to make up our own existential meaning while we wait for the end to come. If that's the story we're living in, shame might be an interesting topic for a discussion, but for the most part it simply plays the role of emotional nausea.

But what if shame is embedded in a story that does have purpose? Even more troubling, what if it is being actively leveraged by the personality of evil to bend us toward sin?

Typically, whenever researchers study and discuss shame, we do so as though it is some abstract emotional or cognitive phenomena. We describe shame as something we would do well to better regulate, but not as an entity that has a conscious will of its own. But I believe we live in a world in which good and evil are not just events that happen to us but rather expressions of something or someone whose *intention* is for good or for evil. And I will suggest that shame is used with this intention to dismantle us as individuals and communities, and destroy all of God's creation. You may not agree, but even so I believe this book will still be helpful for you.

This, then, is a book about the story of shame. The one we tell about it, the one it tells about us, and even more so the one God has been telling about all of us from the beginning. Most important, this book also examines how the story of the Bible offers us a way not only to understand shame but also to effectively put it to death, even if that takes a lifetime to accomplish. But putting shame to death is not simply about addressing it as a deeply destructive emotional and relational nuisance. For we cannot speak of shame without speaking of creation and God's intention for it. From the beginning it has been God's purpose for this world to be one of emerging goodness, beauty and joy. Evil has wielded shame as a primary weapon to see to it that that world never happens. Consequently, to combat shame is not merely to wrestle against something we detest. It is to do that very thing that provides the necessary space for each of us to live like God, become like Jesus and grow up to be who we were born to be.

The premise of this book, then, is that shame is not just a consequence of something our first parents did in the Garden of Eden. It is the emotional weapon that evil uses to (1) corrupt our relationships with God and each other, and (2) disintegrate any and all gifts of vocational vision and creativity. These gifts include any area of endeavor that promotes goodness, beauty and joy in and for the lives of others, whether that be teaching our first graders, loving our spouse well, managing forests, conducting healing prayer services, creating a new medical technology, offering psychotherapy or composing symphonies. Shame is a primary means to prevent us from using the gifts we have been given. And those gifts enable us to flourish as a light-bearing community of Jesus followers who work to create space for others who wish to join it to do so. Shame, therefore, is not simply an unfortunate, random, emotional event that came with us out of the primordial evolutionary soup. It is both a source and result of evil's active assault on God's creation, and a way for evil to try to hold out until the new heaven and earth appear at the consummation of history.

However, while this book holds shame to be within the context of a grand story, and so takes on its place and meaning, within that story's purpose lie the mechanics of how shame works. Familiarity with those mechanisms, through the lens of interpersonal neurobiology, though not substantiating shame's teleology, can open up ways for us to align ourselves with the purpose that God has for a world in which mercy and justice reign, a world teeming with goodness and beauty, and in which joy of true relationship is our destiny.

## A Tale of What Is Ahead

Toward that end, this book approaches our topic as follows. In chapter one I will establish a working description of shame and what we assume it to mean for our purposes. I will describe how we generally experience it and what its nature tends to be in everyday life. Chapters two and three engage our quarry from an interpersonal neurobiological (IPNB) approach. We will take a tour of what the mind is and what it means to flourish from an IPNB perspective, followed by an introduction to how shame operates as a disintegrating force within the mind, relationships and communities.

This sets the stage for chapter four, which reminds us that at our core we are storytelling creatures. To know your story is to know shame's place in it. Here we will explore some features of stories in general, how we tell them and the value of knowing which story you believe you are living in. We will see shame's potential both as cause and effect of the stories we construct. Chapter five invites us specifically into the biblical narrative, offering one way of considering shame in light of the story that followers of Jesus believe they occupy. We consider how in the Genesis account of creation, shame is featured as something that evil has been wielding from the very beginning to corrupt God's intended creation of goodness and beauty.

Chapter six introduces us to the fulcrum on which the healing of shame hangs in the balance. We will discuss the deep reality of what it means that (1) we are relational and therefore necessarily vulnerable beings, and (2) the healing of shame begins and ends in the experience of being known, a biblical notion that begins in the heart of God, is offered to humans in Genesis, and reaches its culmination on Good Friday. Healing shame requires our being vulnerable with other people in embodied actions. There is no other way, but shame will, as we will see, attempt to convince us otherwise.

Chapter seven offers a model for what it means to directly address shame in concrete ways. Passages from the epistle to the Hebrews and the Gospel of John will serve as guides for implementing the requirements necessary for us to not only heal shame but to begin to see how its redemption leads to greater relational integration and opportunity for creative endeavor. Chapter eight then extends the path of what we learn in chapter seven into the primary communities in which we are nurtured: our family, the church and our educational institutions. We will see how these realms have their particular ways of incubating shame, and what we can explicitly do to re-imagine our stories in these most formative of settings.

This brings us to the book's culmination in chapter nine, in which we will explore how shame's healing leads to renewed vitality in the multiple ways God has called us. For in our deliverance from shame we are not simply liberated to be nicer, happier people; rather, we are redeemed to live into those multiple roles of calling—from parenting to teaching to engineering—with joyful creativity.

Reading this book will require varying degrees of effort, for any number of reasons. Combating shame requires more work than you might imagine. I say this not because I am in any way impressed with what is written here or how it has been said; it's not as if the ideas are original to me, for they certainly aren't. Nor do I say it because I have slain all my dragons of shame—far from it. Rather, it is just the opposite. I am deeply aware of how difficult it is to directly confront this problem. I am living proof of this. In fact, the very act of writing this book has revealed more spaces within my inner life that shame inhabits than I would like to admit. The process has activated a whole host of feelings that include fears of inadequacy, worries that I will not be clear or correct or effective, concerns that whatever I may have to say, someone else could say it better, more simply and certainly not require the reader to work so hard to get through all the ink on the paper. I didn't expect that writing a book on shame would be the very thing that revealed just how deeply rooted shame is in me. But frankly, if putting shame to death requires this much hard work, I would rather have folks along for the journey who are willing to do the same, reminding me that I am not alone in the process.

## A FEW CAVEATS

In this book I do not address the distinctives that pertain to shame cultures, shame-honor cultures or shame societies vis-à-vis guilt cultures. Much has been published on these topics, and they are not unhelpful in providing a window through which we can understand societal behavior.

Suffice it to say, however we choose to talk about cultures as a whole, each one has its own particular way of manifesting shame and guilt. These words symbolize human experience that is universal, although certainly the socialization of these fundamental emotional states is bound to shape how we interpret them. These categories of shame-honor and guilt cultures do not imply, either, that shame cultures do not know about or experience the phenomenon of guilt, or that guilt cultures do not experience shame. In this book we are exploring shame not as a socially constructed finding but rather an interpersonal neurobiological event. This is not to say that what you find here is the last word on shame or the only or even the best way to comprehend it. Rather, this is hopefully one way to approach it such that we may live more fully integrated lives.

On another front, I do not address to what degree shame is a good thing, something that we require in society to ensure that people will behave appropriately. In this book I am not debating this question, nor in any way suggesting that all shame experience is necessarily bad. Indeed, it is reasonable to assume that shame as an interpersonal neurobiological process plays a necessary role in helping us develop proper self-regulatory behavior. However, it is equally true that many behaviors that are *not* deterred (but that we believe should be) emerge from established shame-based patterns of life that precede said behaviors. It is beyond the scope of this book to explore every aspect of our topic. My intention here is to address those universal experiences of shame that lead to disintegrated states of mind that end in disintegrated communities with little creative capacity for goodness and beauty.

Still, questions may remain. Exploring in the way I propose, might we not run the risk of dismissing the necessary, helpful aspects of shame too easily? Without it, won't we devolve into madness? Moreover, is there not a clear difference between the shame felt by a woman who commits adultery and a woman who is raped?

Although these are not unimportant questions, they are not the primary subject of our inquiry, nor is there space in this volume to address all of the questions that our topic invariably raises. However, a world in which shame did not exist would also be one in which those very behaviors we fear would be unleashed would not likely exist either, given how many of them emerge out of shame in the first place. And, yes, the story of an adulteress is quite different from that of a rape victim. But the shame that the victim of sexual assault feels is often no more easily healed than that of a woman involved in an affair "simply" because the former "knows" her shame was not a result of her actions. For indeed shame's power lies not so much in facts that we can clarify but rather in its emotional state, which is so much harder to shake.

Throughout this book you will read the stories of people like you and me who are wrestling with shame and doing their best to fix their eyes on Jesus, do what he did and despise it on the way to being liberated to create as they were so intended from the beginning. No matter if you are one who is simply curious about shame or find yourself buried underneath it, I believe this book can offer help and hope.

I acknowledged earlier that you may be either unfamiliar with or do not believe the story the Bible tells. Well, you're in good company. There are many days that I have a hard time believing it myself. The very nature of the world is such that at times it takes near Herculean effort to maintain the conviction that Jesus is real, that God is truly loving and that we are at war with evil. This book, therefore, is no proof text about anything. It is, rather, an invitation to be known, to be loved (whether you believe in God or not), but also to join me and others to risk all you have on a God who would rather die than let anything come between us all. As you read this invitation, then, you may find some practical help for dealing with shame (especially as you apply the elements of IPNB), even if the big story of the Bible doesn't yet feel comfortable enough to try on. At the very least I'll be glad to know that in having read this book you have found yourself to be drawn into relationships that are more joyful and intimate, engaged in work that is more meaningful and creative, and casting a vision for seeing goodness and beauty where perhaps before you did not.

At the book's conclusion you will find questions associated with each chapter for further discussion. Shame is not something we "fix" in the privacy of our mental processes; evil would love for us to believe that to be so. We combat it within the context of conversation, prayer and other communal, embodied actions. Therefore I encourage you to use the questions not only for your own personal use but also for engaging one another as a means of healing in real time and space.

With these thoughts in mind, I invite you to join me in discovering the soul of shame, the story it is trying to tell and the alternative story of goodness and beauty that God is telling, one that God is imagining for us all, one in which he is doing "immeasurably more than all we ask or imagine, according to his power that is at work within us."

# 1

# Our Problem with Shame

No, I'm not willing to do that." He was succinct and clear. I inquired what he felt as he imagined telling his wife about the affair. "Terrified." Of what, I asked? He could only describe in vague terms the abject sense of humiliation he would have to endure should this illicit relationship come to light.

●●●

She was the chief executive of a successful marketing firm and had relied on her hard-driving style to get things done. She was bewildered that her company was listing, and her effort to work harder was not effectively righting the ship. She was running out of ideas. I inquired as to whom she could ask for help. Without hesitation she informed me that to admit she needed assistance was tantamount to resigning. "I can't afford not to have ideas that work. If I have to ask for help, I will be seen as incompetent and the board will fire me."

●●●

"She didn't get in, and I'm worried about what this will mean for her future." This, coming from a mother who had worked diligently to do her part to help her daughter gain entrance to her top school choice. This might be understandable, except for the fact that her daughter was only three years old.

●●●

Why had no one protected her? By the time she was twenty-six she had slept with over fifteen men and endured two abortions. But the sex had begun when she was eleven, with an uncle who had first treated her as special, but eventually threatened her very life if she were to reveal the horror. This lasted until she was seventeen, when she left for college, where she was free of her uncle but imprisoned to the behavior that was the only path she knew to "intimacy" with a man. How in the world was she to tell her parents, let alone friends or anyone in her faith community? The only reason she was telling me was that her depression had become too overwhelming for her to function.

●●●

The hypothesis had finally been proven. The elegant biochemistry, the complex statistical analysis of the patients' clinical responses to the drug, and a little luck had all added up. All the work, all the long hours away from his family, all the grant money spent—it was all finally worth it. Along with this discovery would certainly come the offer of a tenured position he had long coveted and that the university would be unable to deny him. Not to mention the potential earnings once the patent came through. There was only one problem. An ethics board that was tasked to make sure his lab's research was beyond reproach had found some questionable data reporting. And before the week was over, his life was unraveling faster than he could have imagined, the result of someone's need to make history fighting cancer.

●●●

He began drinking when he was thirteen. He had two DUIs by the time he was twenty, the second one landing him in jail for a month. That was more than two decades ago, before he met Jesus. But in the last five years the bourbon had begun to flow again most evenings after everyone went to bed. His wife had informed him that if the drinking didn't stop, she was leaving and taking the children with her. Then there was the issue of his work. How, exactly, would he tell the people of his congregation where he had been the pastor for fifteen years? Jim Beam seemed to be the only thing that helped him hang on in the face of the burnout he felt shepherding such a challenging flock.

## OUR STORIES OF SHAME

Stories. Each of us has one, and at some point the people in the previous scenarios sat in my office telling me his or hers. And theirs are just the tip of the iceberg. There are many more, each with different screenplays, each that emerges from a different family of origin, each with its own particular joys and sorrows, victories and defeats. No matter what initially brings them to see me, their stories eventually lead to the moment when what I believe to be the lowest common denominator in human relationships makes its way into the room. It matters not if the person earns a two-comma salary or works for minimum wage. She may be married or single. He may be African American or Caucasian. Depressed, anxious or just plain angry; happy, sad or indifferent. He may be the father or the son, the employer or employee. It may be an individual, a couple, family, community, school or business organization. And you needn't have ever darkened the office door of a psychiatrist. It doesn't require the breakdown of our mental health to be plagued with it. It only requires that you have a pulse. To be human is to be infected with this phenomenon we call shame.

Shame is something we all experience at some level, more consciously for some than for others. Of course there are the obvious examples that come to mind: times we have felt everything from slight embarrassment to deep humiliation. The tabloids are rife with cover stories of the latest follies of celebrities or politicians who have behaved badly. But many of us carry shame less publicly, often outside the easy view of even some of our closest friends. Unemployment. Having a family member whose alcoholism is displayed in front of your friends. Losing a major account at work. The breakup of a marriage. Our child's seeming disinterest in school. A boss whose motivational tactic is to regularly compare your work to that of someone else who is outperforming you. Any of these more common scenarios carry the burden of shame in ways that we work hard to cover up. And our coping strategies have become so automatic that we may be completely unaware of its presence and activity.

Shame can vary in its range from the most relationally subtle ways—the condescending glance or tone of voice from one spouse to another—to wholesale cultural movements that involve groups, communities and eventually nations that war against nations—the biblical story of Dinah in Genesis 34, racial bigotry and suppression, or the murder of a woman for having publicly shamed her family, known commonly in some cultures as an honor killing. It is therefore not merely a function of the things I think or say about myself or others, nor is it limited to what happens between two individuals. It can move stealthily from the bedroom or kitchen to the playing field to the boardroom to the Situation Room, where decisions are made on a global scale. In this way, even the slightest shaming interactions between individuals can eventually grow into conflagrations that involve multiple parties. Longstanding conflicts such as those in the Middle East or East Los Angeles are evidence that when individuals do not address the shame they experience at a personal level, the potential kindling effect can eventually engulf whole regions of humanity. One of the purposes of this book is to emphasize that what we do with shame on an individual level has potentially geometric consequences for any of the social systems we occupy, be that our family, place of employment, church or larger community.

It is also important at the outset of this book to note that I do not consider this infestation to be neutral or benign. This is not merely a felt emotion that eventually morphs into words such as "I'm bad." As I will suggest, this phenomenon is the primary tool that evil leverages, out of which emerges everything that we would call sin. As such, it is actively, *intentionally*, at work both within and between individuals. Its goal is to disintegrate any and every system it targets, be that one's personal story, a family, marriage, friendship, church, school, community, business or political system. Its power lies in its subtlety and its silence, and it will not be satisfied until all hell breaks loose. Literally.

Over the last ten years I have been privileged to walk with people as they have been courageously engaging their stories, moving to places of greater depth and connection with God and others while applying new insights that have emerged from the field of interpersonal neurobiology, which I explore in *Anatomy of the Soul*. They have learned about various

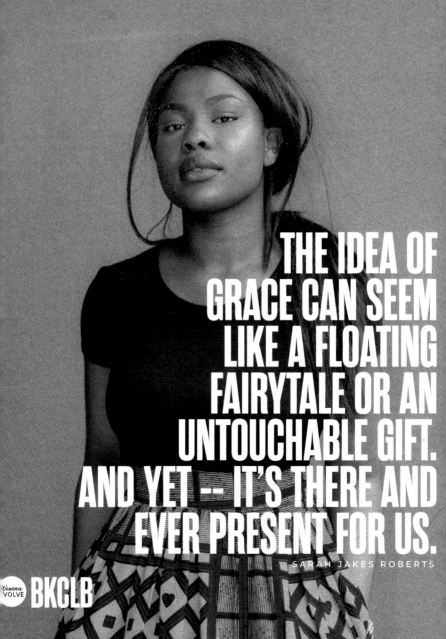

THE IDEA OF GRACE CAN SEEM LIKE A FLOATING FAIRYTALE OR AN UNTOUCHABLE GIFT. AND YET -- IT'S THERE AND EVER PRESENT FOR US.

SARAH JAKES ROBERTS

BKCLB

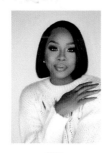

*Sis,*

I've gotten to the point that I don't back down from many things. It's less about trusting who I am and wholly knowing that I am limitless because of who I serve. It's just that simple. I've seen what happens when we lean into and grab hold of the power of God -- literal miracles, signs and wonders. Perhaps there was a time that I did cower under the weight of opposition, when it was harder to see myself as God does. But these days, at the mere whisper of an enemy's lie, I'm ready to square up. And that's on, no weapon formed against me shall ever prosper, ok?

But I know what it's like to be tempted. When our pasts and the decisions we've made created a story that didn't align with God's best, or when the aftermath of an exposed secret hovers in the dark corners of our lives, we can run from every opportunity to tell a different narrative about who we really are. The idea of grace can seem like a floating fairytale or an untouchable gift. And yet -- it's there and ever present for us. What a beautiful and generous God we serve.

One thing about us around WEBC? Chilllle, we won't perish for lack of knowledge. These reading journeys are to teach us and equip us. We're learning the language and tools that enable us to partner with God in our own freedom and stand surely in the telling of our testimony. So we read and we share and we grow together. This month is no different.

The Soul of Shame, our May book, is as much a learning resource as it is a Spirit-breathed tool in helping us develop a system to overcome the threat of shame in our lives. Its incredible author, Curt Thompson is an educated and licensed psychiatrist who, through the lens of Jesus, provides us with insights about how the brain affects and processes trauma and relationships, all aimed to help people discover a fresh perspective and practical applications to foster healthy and vibrant lives, allowing them to get unstuck and move toward the next beautiful thing they're being called to make.

There is an assignment attached to each of our lives. Powerful, life-giving, world shaking assignments. God said it and I believe it! And if I do nothing else, I will stand at the ready to ensure that we can actualize them and bring the Kingdom to earth, one woman at a time.

Are you with me?

*Sarah Jakes Roberts*

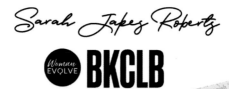

domains of the mind and what it means to love God and others with all of it. They have realized what it means to pay attention to what they pay attention to; the overarching role of emotion in human activity; how memory is as much about predicting the future as it is about recalling the past; how their patterns of attachments with their primary caregivers and current intimate relationships shape their experiences of God; that our awareness of God's deep, joyful pleasure with us at all times everywhere changes everything about how we interpret what we sense, image, feel, think and do; that life is not about not being messy but about being creative with the messes we have; that ruptures will occur but resilience and life is to be found in how we repair them; and that Jesus has come not only to show us how to do all of the aforementioned but to empower us to do so on the way to God's kingdom coming in its fullness.

All this has been very good news for many. However, invariably, on the way to greater freedom they must pass, as we all do, through a common place of suffering: the place of shame. It may be cloaked in the minute details of one's narrative or on public display. It may be obscured in the language of other emotions we are more familiar with such as sadness, anger, disappointment or even guilt. Or it may be a deeply, consciously felt presence in many of our waking hours. We may have different events, images, words or explicit feelings that represent it. It may be consumptive or we may barely notice its activity in our day-to-day comings and goings. Eventually, however, we all come face to face with this specter, the (virtually) unspoken, primal obstacle to our growth and flourishing, and it seems there is no getting around it.

What then exactly is this thing we are calling shame? How do we distinguish it in the moment it occurs? From the countless hours spent with people on their respective pilgrimages, it seems that even defining it is no easy task, which, as I will invite you to consider later, is part of shame's intention. For its elusiveness is a key element of its power. We can use various words such as *humiliation, embarrassment, indignity, disgrace* or more. And though these words get close to what we really mean, ultimately they are essentially symbols that represent the actual *neuropsychological state* we enter when we experience it.

It is not easy to wrap a simple classification or explanation around our topic. However, despite the challenge of developing such a universally accepted definition of shame, there are particular qualities about it that we immediately recognize as being common to our experience of it.

## More Than a Feeling

One way to approach its essence is to understand it as an undercurrent of sensed emotion, of which we may have either a slight or robust impression that, should we put words to it, would declare some version of *I am not enough*; *There is something wrong with me*; *I am bad*; or *I don't matter*.

But we would be mistaken if we thought that the story of shame begins with those words or that they tell it in its entirety. For although we come to understand much of who we are via the medium of language as a way to make sense of reality, our lives emerge most primally in the forms of bodily sensations and movements, perceptions, and emotions. Emotion itself could be considered to be the gasoline in our human tank. If we were to take emotion out of the human experience, we would literally stop moving. Hence, although the description of our experience of shame is often couched in words, its essence is first felt. Though I may say, "I should have been better at that" or "I'm not good enough," the power of those moments lies in our emotional response to the evoking stimulus, be that a comment, a glance or a recollection of that day in third grade when your teacher pointed out in front of the rest of the class that you weren't that bright.

We use many different words to convey various bandwidths of emotional tone. We know that pleasure and sadness are different, that disappointment and anger are not felt to be the same. But it is revealing that so many of what we would term "negative" emotions (i.e., those that we find generally to be distressing in some way) are actually rooted in shame. Again, by shame I am not talking about something that necessarily requires the intensity of extreme humiliation. Rather, it is born out of a sense of "there being something wrong" with me or of "not being enough," and therefore exudes the aroma of being unable or powerless to change one's condition or circumstances.

The important feature here is not just the *fact* that I am not enough to change my life (though of course the fact is necessary as part of the experience), but rather the *felt sense that I do not have what it takes to tolerate this moment or circumstance*. There are other examples of this. Qualitatively, we would not usually associate sadness with shame. If I lose my best friend to cancer, I do not initially anticipate that shame would be anywhere close to what I would feel. But sadness, though certainly not always, is often related to a lessening. A lessening of relationship (such as death or a betrayal), function or agency (unemployment or an amputation), or the nature of one's story (discovering as an adult, for instance, that when you were a child your father had had an affair and fathered a child you have never known about, lessening the confidence you have in your place in your family). In each case, we inevitably encounter the moment when we are not enough to change our reality as we are currently imagining it. As such, this "not being enough" to tolerate this moment is the grounding for how shame operates, albeit in dimensions of mental activity that may escape my immediate awareness of it as shame.

The purpose here is not to prove that all emotion that we experience as uncomfortable is rooted in shame, but that we notice many of the emotions that represent distress within us are an extended development of this particular emotional state. Out of this state, then, arise words that we use to make sense of it, so that we can do something about it. When Alison brought her test result to her mother showing a score of 92 percent, her mother asked, "What happened to the other 8 percent?" It doesn't take much to imagine what Alison sensed and felt, nor would it be a surprise if you were to learn that in the wake of multiple interactions like this one Alison developed a knack for telling herself (among many possible options) that she simply had not worked hard enough. Furthermore, she would go on to tell herself that she needed to work harder in order to improve her scores. She would not necessarily be aware that such self-talk was primarily about coping with shame, despite this being the most fundamental thing she is doing. And so, out of the feelings of shame come the words *I don't work hard enough.*

However, soon enough, the words we use double back to reinforce the feelings. Alison, by repeatedly telling herself that she is never working hard enough (and therefore needs to work harder) deepens the felt sensation of shame. Hence, an unending loop is created: sensations and feelings beget thoughts that in turn strengthen the felt experience. And so we see that shame is certainly formed in the world of emotion, but it eventually recruits and involves our thinking, imaging and behaving as well.

Thus, from the outset we come to the realization that shame is both ubiquitous in its presence (there is no person or experience it does not taint) and infinitely shape-shifting in its presentation. If it were a member of the Periodic Table of elements, it might be carbon, the element common to all living organisms. That it is so fundamental within our existence also makes it quite challenging to root out. If we approach it as a problem that we can solve merely by changing how or what we think, we are likely to limit our effectiveness in combating it. This is what Matt discovered.

As a marketing executive he had developed a successful business and now had several employees working for him. He was conscientious and cared about his workers, treating them generously and justly. But he worried that at any moment the economy would shift enough that he would have to lay someone off or, worse, that the business would fail outright, which at times kept him up at night. He was insightful enough to recognize that he could not control all the variables that determined whether his company would survive; furthermore, he easily admitted that he worried too much about, well, just about everything. He came for help because he saw his problem primarily as one of anxiety; it was not debilitating but present enough to get his wife's attention. It was not making sense to her (and eventually to him) that despite the steady progression of his business, Matt sometimes would find himself ruminating about how he and his family would one day end up living in a box under a bridge. One noteworthy caveat was how effectively he compartmentalized all of this. Anyone who knew him, apart from his wife, would never have guessed that he had a care in the world, as he had practiced how to effectively manage his concerns when in the presence of just about everyone, ironically, because as he would later tell me, he worried about what people would think of him if they knew about how much he worried. Go figure.

He came to see me to explore the possibility of using cognitive therapy to restructure his thinking about his life. This was a reasonable goal, as cognitive-based interventions have been demonstrated to be effective in treating a number of emotional problems, especially anxiety. But despite Matt's best efforts, he continued to feel wrapped around the axle of an imagined catastrophic future. One of the most glaring troubles for him was the reality that his life with God did not seem to be able to budge his incessant trend toward ruminating about disaster. Despite the fact that his relationship with Jesus was the most important thing in his life, thinking and reflecting on Scripture passages that admonished him to leave anxiety at the door only left him standing at the door's threshold, right along with his worry. For him, it was not until we began to explore the nature of his experience as one that was *felt*, *sensed* and *imaged* as much as it was *thought* that he began to gain some traction in overcoming his problem.

For instance, we quickly uncovered that what he felt as worry was often correlated with thoughts such as *I won't be able to figure out what to do if the work starts to drop off.* (This, despite his having navigated effectively more than one downturn in business over the course of his career.) Or even more commonly he found himself thinking, *Sooner or later I'm going to be found out to be the fraud I am.* He agreed that most of his friends would find his way of thinking hard to fathom, given his consistent history of competence. Matt's interest was in confronting these thoughts with alternative thinking processes. This is standard operating procedure for cognitive-behavioral therapy. But in his case we found that despite his best effort at restructuring his thinking, this approach still left him with the residual *feeling* that undergirded the thought *I do not have what it takes. When it will count most, I will not be enough.*

On the surface of Matt's complaint, it appeared that his primary problem was one of anxiety, and surely anxiety was a problem. But further exploration revealed that under all of this was a deep *sense* that he simply did not have what it took to be effective, a sensation that was not reducible to a statement but rather something that seemed to have been woven into his DNA. Although we often try to get our minds around shame by using language (which is not unimportant), its essence precedes language; we

therefore often have difficulty regulating it by using words. Telling ourselves we shouldn't be ashamed often only reinforces it.

## JUDGE NOT LEST YE BE JUDGED

One of the hallmarks of shame is its employment of judgment. Here, by
*judgment* I am not referring to the necessary, everyday process of discernment required by each of us for navigating our lives wisely. Nor am
I considering the actions taken by maturing, flourishing people to set
appropriate limits for themselves or others, be that within a family,
church, business or government. Rather, I am referring to the spirit of
condemnation or condescension with which we analyze or critique
something, whether ourselves or someone or something else. I may say
to myself, *I should have done better at that assignment.* What is crucial is
the emotional tone that undergirds those words. The spirit of judgment
Jesus warned against is such a common part of our mental lives that we
barely notice its presence. In fact, it can become so automatic that its
manifestation does not require spoken words but rather presents as
something felt. Nor is it necessary to be overtly harsh; indeed, much of
what passes as "reasonable observations" about ourselves or others is
merely cloaked judgment.

Will believed he knew how to get the most out of his employees, which
was to regularly point out their shortcomings so as to "encourage" improvement. He was unaware that his constant criticism was one of the
reasons there was such a high turnover rate in his company. He had
always assumed that people simply were either unwilling to work hard
or to accept honest feedback. It never occurred to him that his penchant
for managing people in this way was rooted in his own sense of inadequacy and shame, which he had learned to cope with by turning it
outward toward others.

Parents experience a similar result when we have to discipline our
children, especially our teenagers, whom we believe we can reason with
by the use of our impeccable logic (letting them know that ours is patently obvious and theirs is groundless). We believe we are merely correcting their actions, but fail to see that in offering what we consider to

be necessary measures, shame enters the process. We are perplexed at why they don't respond to our logical arguments for why they shouldn't be smoking pot or hooking up with their friends.

But it is important to be aware that the act of judging others has its origins in our self-judgment. As I often tell patients, "Shamed people shame people." Long before we are criticizing others, the source of that criticism has been planted, fertilized and grown in our own lives, directed at ourselves, and often in ways we are mostly unaware of. Suffice to say that our self-judgment, that tendency to tell ourselves that we are not enough—not thin enough, not smart enough, not funny enough, not . . . enough—is the nidus out of which grows our judgment of others, not least being our judgment of God. The problem is that we have constructed a sophisticated lattice of blindness around this behavior, which disallows our awareness of it.

Eventually, judgment, and the shame that is its master, can become the source of an ever-enlarging circle of conflict. We have all had experiences in which someone's criticism of another, even though subtle at first, expands to include additional people until whole systems are involved and corrupted by it. Soon enough, what started out as Mary's stated opinion about Stan's proposal during the school board meeting devolved into entire groups of people publicly choosing sides not just about how to spend several thousand dollars but privately about personalities, with anger and hurt strewn everywhere in its wake. It doesn't take much to make the jump to how these forms of conflict, writ large on the community or world stage, lead to the violence we see all around us.

## HIDE AND SEEK

Another feature of shame's presentation is that of hiding. Whether it is the involution into the silence of our own minds or the literal turning away from someone with a downcast facial expression with eyes lowered, shame leads us to cloak ourselves with invisibility to prevent further intensification of the emotion. It is not hard to bring to mind a secret you have worked hard to keep as a countermeasure against the rejection you anticipate you will have to endure should someone find out the truth about you. The expense of this labor is often buried as hidden cost, as we collect multiple secrets and keep them neatly stacked in our closets—until the closet can no longer contain them.

This clandestine behavior manifests across the entire spectrum of what we would generally consider to be noble or ignoble activity. We can be a felon or a Rhodes Scholar. In either case we will have elements of our life that are expressions of shame, hidden in our embezzlement *or* our appointment to the Federal Court of Appeals bench. Stephen's diligent work was certainly a tribute to his devotion to having spent hours honing his skill as a trial lawyer. But after his marriage began to crumble under the weight of having committed far less energy to his wife and children than to his clients, he was brought up short. Although judged by his peers to be unsurpassed in his profession, he eventually was willing to admit that a great deal of his work was energized by his longstanding worry of being found out to be wrong. Wrong about a case. Wrong about his choice of profession. Wrong about his ideas about politics or theology. Wrong about his ideas about God. He recounted how growing up his family dinner table conversations, ostensibly couched merely as playful verbal jousting, became his father's opportunity to criticize his ideas—all in the name of needing to make sure Stephen's thinking was sound about everything. Eventually this gave birth to not only a way of studying but also living in general that made the management of feeling "not smart enough" his number one emotional priority. Given his otherwise amiable and kind demeanor, no one would have guessed the degree to which he covertly lived in the midst of his shame.

Gloria spent thirty years of marriage to a man she loved before coming to terms with the abortion she had had as a teenager—but had never revealed to her husband. Not until she found herself on the brink of a psychiatric implosion did she begin to consider her history. It is standard practice for me to inquire in the very first session with patients about their sexual history, or if they have endured any significant sexual, physical or emotional trauma as they understand it. Despite this, it was not until I had been seeing Gloria for about two months that she was finally able to tell her story, as if she had been unaware of it at the time of our first encounter. As the veterans of Alcoholics Anonymous report, we are only as sick as the secrets we keep. And shame is committed to keeping us sick.

## CAUGHT IN THE LOOP

We recognize early and often that shame tends to be self-reinforcing. When we experience shame, we tend to turn away from others because the prospect of being seen or known by another carries the anticipation of shame being intensified or reactivated. However, the very act of turning away, while temporarily protecting and relieving us from our feeling (and the gaze of the "other"), ironically simultaneously reinforces the very shame we are attempting to avoid. Notably, we do not necessarily realize this to be happening—we're just trying to survive the moment. But indeed this dance between hiding and feeling shame itself becomes a tightening of the noose. We feel shame, and then feel shame for feeling shame. It begets itself.

Athletic and attractive, no one would have suspected it of her at first glance. Nancy had been bingeing and purging for the better part of fifteen years. She had kept it a secret rather effectively from the time she was a teenager until she was into her first year of marriage. When her husband, Mark, first discovered it, he immediately suggested they both seek professional help, but she stonewalled. He was stunned at this skeleton in her closet, given how well he thought they had worked at being honest in their communication heading into marriage. Now he simply felt helpless to do anything about it. Every time he raised his concern, Nancy firmly, and sometimes harshly, redirected the conversation, indicating that the very act of talking about it unleashed an unbearable torrent of shame, which made it impossible for her to even look at him. And so she turned away. Away from Mark, away from the immediacy of the sensation of shame and toward the very behaviors that would only increase the burden of shame she carried over time. Every time this cycle repeated itself, every time she attempted to deflect her shame by turning, she revolved into an ever more tightly spun spool of that which she was hoping to avoid becoming.

## DIVIDE AND CONQUER

Isolation and disconnection are natural consequences of hiding and re-
sisting reengagement. With enough reinforcement of the features we have
thus far considered, we see how the outcome is the separation of people
from one another. In any of the previous examples, relational disintegration
is obvious. But this isolation is not limited to that between people. For as
we will see in chapter two, the fundamental neurobiology of the experience
of shame disintegrates different neural networks and their corresponding
functions within each individual brain, isolating them, causing the mind to
be decreasingly flexible in its capacity to adapt to its environment. In order
for us to flourish, we need to be able to connect with others, but this connection is deeply rooted in our ongoing work to increase the degree of
connection we experience within our own minds. As Daniel Siegel and
others have pointed out, this process of intra- and interpersonal integration
is a dance that depends on the fluid movement between the work of the
individual and that of a community.[1] I need the community in order for my
mind to be integrated, and with a more integrated mind I will be more able
to work toward a more integrated community, which reinforces the cycle.
Shame both actively dismantles and further prohibits this process of integration, leading to disconnection between mental processes within an individual's mind as well as between individual members within a community.

As a child and adolescent Helen had never considered her family to
be broken. It never struck her as odd that her older brother, Jack, consistently received attention from her parents (especially her mother) that
she did not. She simply attributed it to the fact that he had been the
golden boy of their local school and church community; his reward was
well-deserved. Her parents were quick to publicly shower accolades on
him but offered nary a mention of her. This pattern continued into
adulthood; even when Helen and Jack were married and had children of
their own, Jack's children received particular affection, which Helen's did
not. Her response was simply to work harder to gain her parents' affirmation, now for her children as much as for herself.

Eventually it all became too much. During one family reunion when
the conversation again turned naturally to all that Jack had been accom-

plishing at his work, and then moved to his son's new interest in baseball, Helen, longing to be seen, offered how delighted she had been at her daughter's interest in lacrosse. She might as well have been speaking to an empty chair. Her mother, ignoring Helen's comment, asked what position Jack's son liked to play. No one was prepared for what happened next.

It began with the slinging of a plate of food and the breaking of a wine glass. Her tirade erupted and continued for ten uninterrupted minutes, with forty years of neglect and hurt spewing over anyone within earshot and sightline. It only stopped when the emotional ammunition chamber was empty. She and her husband left without waiting for a response from her brother or parents. Predictably, in the aftermath and attempted cleanup of the brouhaha, her parents said nothing about the past forty years or the role they played in it. They only had words for the last ten minutes Helen spent at the reunion and all of the trouble she had caused. They expected her to make things right, and especially with her brother. Of course.

Helen's story reflects how the shame of emotional neglect, even and perhaps particularly because of how unremarkable it seemed in the early years of her life, led to her feeling isolated and cut off from her family. Eventually this led to an event in which the whole system was disintegrating. Given shame's intention to provoke the process of isolation, neither Helen nor her family system had the wherewithal to repair the toxic rupture.

In all these features of shame, emotion is at the heart of the matter; judgment is actively in play. In their hiding, people become disconnected from each other and within their own minds, and the process tends to snowball, caught in a self-perpetuating loop. Is there hope for us? Fortunately, there remains one response to shame that can begin to point us in the right direction.

## OUR COUNTERINTUITIVE CONFLICT

With little effort we can get a sense of how the essential feeling of shame would lead to judging, hiding, reinforcement and isolation. It is not so straightforward to see that exposure is the very thing that shame requires for healing. Given how compelled we feel to turn away, strike inward at ourselves or strike out at others in response to shame, it is not our intuition to then quickly turn *toward the other* as a means to resolve the problem. When we are in the middle of a shame storm, it feels virtually impossible to turn again to see the face of someone, even someone we might otherwise feel safe with. It is as if our only refuge is in our isolation; the prospect of exposing what we feel activates our anticipation of further shame.

The work required to overcome the inertia of shame and turn in a posture of vulnerability toward someone else can initially feel overwhelming. Later, we will consider tactics for beginning this process in earnest. But it is helpful to remember that part of shame's power lies in its ability to isolate, both within and between minds. The very thing that has the power to heal this emotional nausea is the reunion of those parts of us that have been separated.

The school system in which Jordan had grown up prided itself in the number of gifted and talented programs it provided for elementary and middle school children, and then the number of AP courses it offered its high school students. What had started out as an attempt to provide more opportunity for students, however, eventually devolved into a cauldron of pressure and anxiety for students and parents alike. Instead of providing an opportunity for expanding curiosity and deepening character, teachers wound up being caught in the same vortex, feeling the pressure to train their students to score well on AP exams so they could get in the best colleges. No longer was school and the learning it represented joy filled. Instead it had become a factory of worry. Worry that was fueled by shame. The institutional shame that the school and all of its parts—test scores, students, teachers and administrators—carried was subtle but palpable. All driven by the fear that no matter how many graduating seniors were admitted to Ivy League universities, they would eventually be judged and found wanting.

By the time Jordan had finished graduate school and had begun his work as a high school English teacher, he wanted life for his students to be different from what it had been for him. And so he began inviting his students to a local coffee shop gathering once a month after school for conversations about what it was like to be in their place in life. They talked about a range of topics, but eventually the discussion turned to how much pressure they felt and how worried they were about their performance, not only in his class but in just about everything they were engaged in. They described how alone they felt in their worry. Life for them wasn't very joyful, but they figured this was the price they had to pay to get into the right college so they could find the right job so they could make the right amount of money so they could start the whole process over again with their own kids. But of significance was that some students spoke of how hard, even embarrassing, it was to admit to the weight they were under. They described how they believed they should simply be able to survive this pressure cooker, and to complain that something wasn't right about it would make them seem weak. They felt vulnerable talking about it openly, even with Jordan and their friends in what was for them a relatively safe venue.

But what they found to be most helpful—and had them coming back month after month to the coffee shop—was that in admitting their embarrassment, they didn't feel nearly as alone, and many reported over the course of their year that the pressure to perform, and the fear of the shame of not performing well, gradually receded. The connection they experienced with Jordan and each other actually enabled them to feel more at ease as students. Eventually, word got out to administrators about what was happening in these gatherings. The administrators invited Jordan to talk more openly about the conversations, which ultimately led to a restructuring of the curriculum, including a reduction in the number of AP classes offered at the school. This is a rare story in education, but it began with one teacher courageously creating the opportunity for institutional shame to be exposed in the voices of those for whom the school ostensibly existed.

In this example we see how shame's healing encompasses the counterintuitive act of turning toward what we are most terrified of. We fear the shame that we will feel when we speak of that very shame. In some circumstances we anticipate this vulnerable exposure to be so great that it will be almost life threatening. But it is in the *movement toward another*, toward connection with someone who is safe, that we come to know life and freedom from this prison. And in Jordan's story, not just an indi-

vidual but an entire institutional system came to breathe fresh air on its
way to a more integrated state and liberation from shame.

## PILGRIMS ON A JOURNEY

Although it is tempting to hope that we can eliminate shame from our
relational diet, it is futile to wish for this. Our hope is, rather, in changing
our response to it as we journey together toward God's kingdom, which
is now but not yet in its fullness. We would like to have it excised surgi-
cally from our brains, but instead find ourselves having to grow in our
confidence in combating it. To do so requires that we strengthen our
capacity to turn our attention to something other than shame. As such
we do not execute shame quickly via some behavioral guillotine, but
rather we starve it over time, not by avoiding it but by attuning to it as a
component of a larger story. A story whose beginning is as much about
*how* we were made as it is about *why* we were made. Part of that *how* is
the subject of chapter two, a subject that will add a helpful layer of understanding in our pursuit of making sense not only of shame but of the
story that the gospel tells in order to realize its healing.

# How Shame Targets the Mind

Justin had never spoken of this to anyone. Only now, as a bachelor in his late thirties, did he seek help, when the repeated collision between his longing for female companionship and his abject terror of rejection once he became involved with a woman reached its nadir. Despite his overwhelming success, first as an investment broker and then as an entrepreneur, he was convinced that something was quite wrong with him. Why was it that every time he became emotionally close with a woman he genuinely cared for, he began to construct, almost involuntarily, barriers to further connection? Eventually, the pattern would repeat itself and the prophecy would be fulfilled that despite his desire he was not able to have a close relationship with a woman.

It was not long into the course of our psychotherapy work that I once again inquired about his sexual development, including any history of having been sexually mistreated. Justin looked at me blankly. His silence lasted several seconds. Finally he said barely above a whisper, "There was a cousin."

He went on to describe, quite painstakingly, his relationship with this older male relative Justin had deeply admired. When Justin was nine years old, his cousin introduced him to pornography. This eventually led to sexual behavior between them that Justin found to be simultaneously stimulating and arousing as well as repulsive. This form of intimacy lasted for three to four years, and Justin had told no one until his conversation with me. I inquired if he had ever considered telling his parents. Justin had thought that to be out of the question at the time. His confusion and shame about his behavior combined with his cousin's irreproachable standing in the family convinced Justin he would not be believed.

Out of these experiences, however, grew an ever-increasing discomfort with any emotionally close attachment. Any friendships, whether with males or females, quickly began to elicit deep feelings of shame as soon as they moved to more intimate places of being known. I suggested to Justin that exploring the way the brain works might help him to better understand and change his experience of shame that kept him locked in his unending relational pattern of sadness and isolation. What was actually happening neurobiologically within him and between him and others in the course of his repetitive relational patterns? Furthermore, what difference would it make to be familiar with these things?

As it turns out, a great deal; for in better understanding the intended course for the healthy neurobiological and relational development of the mind—and shame's effect on that development—we become more familiar with shame's nature, and thereby are enabled to respond to it in concrete, effective ways. In this way, God provides yet another means within creation (the findings of neuroscience and its related disciplines) that reflects Jesus' redemptive mission, simultaneously pointing to the coming new heaven and earth.[1] And redemption was something Justin desperately needed.

Over the last decade emerging information about the brain has continued to gain the interest of researchers and the lay public alike. Hardly a month goes by that the *New York Times Magazine* does not have an article on what we are learning about the brain, and of the twelve issues of *Scientific American* published in 2012, four featured cover articles addressing some aspect of the mind.[2] (Not to mention *Scientific American*'s bimonthly publication *Scientific American: MIND.*) The shelves are bowing with the new volumes being written about everything from memory to neuroplasticity to mirror neurons—and how knowing more about them affects the way we think about our futures; practice science, ethics, law and education; and make a whole host of public policy decisions.

In *Anatomy of the Soul* I explored interpersonal neurobiology and its intersection with Christian spiritual formation. For a detailed survey of those ideas, I refer you to that volume. Here, I'll provide a review of several elements of what is presented there; bearing them in mind can assist us in our understanding of shame.

## THE MIND: A WORKING DEFINITION

First, the mind—where shame originates and lives—is neither limited to nor should it be understood merely in terms of what or how we *think*. Instead, it is, in the language of interpersonal neurobiology (IPNB), a fluid, emerging process that is both embodied and relational, whose task is to regulate the flow of energy and information.[3] It is a fluid process in that it is literally never completely at rest. We are always sensing, imaging, feeling, thinking or acting out something, whether consciously or unconsciously, while awake or asleep. Furthermore, the mind is emerging. This refers to the idea that the whole activity of the brain is greater than the sum of its parts. As elegant as it is, a neuron by itself can't do much, but put 100 billion of them in concert, albeit different in their individual makeup and function, and before long things begin to happen that one could not easily predict: Dvorak's *New World Symphony*, Van Gogh's *The Mulberry Tree* or the discovery of quantum mechanics. Moreover, not only these seemingly remarkable feats but also "simple" acts of healing, patience, forgiveness, confession and setting healthy limits in relationships demonstrate the mind's emergence. However, the mind equally has the capacity for creating Auschwitz. Emergence, when bent, can amount to hell on earth. As we will see, this is what I suggest is evil's ultimate shame-wielding purpose.

In addition to being fluid and emergent the mind is embodied. It is not some abstraction that exists somewhere in the subjective ether; nor is it merely limited to the brain, but rather via the brain's extended nervous system the mind interacts with the world both inside and outside our skin. We know we are anxious by the nature of our sweaty palms or increased pulse. When we are in love, we do not just love the object of our affections; we love what we feel inside ourselves when we are with or think of him or her. The flutter in our chest. The lightness of our perceived mood. And those feelings are perceived as much as a function of our bodies as anything else. Were it not for our fully embodied experience of our mind, we would be unaware of much of what our mind is trying to tell us.

Furthermore, the mind is as relational as it is embodied. By this I mean that the very emergence of the mind's capacity to do what it does is crucially dependent on the presence of relationships. From the day we enter the world, our neurons are firing not only out of the depths of genetically influenced patterns but also in response to the myriad of social interactions we sense and perceive when we encounter other people. Not only this, but data from the field of epigenetics now suggest that human experience has the capacity to turn genes on and off.[4] In this way, our relational interactions can actually influence our lives at the most basic biological level. Thus, the way our neurological system wires its responses to various emotional experiences is significantly influenced by the relational contexts in which those emotions arise. This means that the "nature versus nurture" boundary is illusory when it comes to the development of the mind.

The task of the mind, in terms of what we witness scientifically that it does most effectively (and not from a theological perspective), is to regulate the flow of energy and information. *Energy* refers to the literal electrochemical communication from neuron to neuron. And *information* refers to those meaningful perceptions, whether conscious or nonconscious, that are coursing through our lives every moment, that are correlated with that very neurobiological energy. Shame has a tendency to disrupt this process of "regulating the flow of energy and information" by effectively disconnecting various functions of the mind from one another, leaving each domain of the mind as cut off from one another as we feel ourselves to be disconnected from other people.

Notice that when speaking of the interaction between energy and information, I do not refer to neurobiological substrates (energy) being causes but rather correlates of the phenomena (information) we experience and process. We must be clear at all times that although the brain and the extensions of the central and autonomic nervous systems are necessary for life, we who follow Jesus do not believe that our minds—and therefore the essence of who *we* "are"—can be reduced to the neuronal activity of the brain. Thus, when we feel anger, imagine the Grand Canyon, cheer for our favorite soccer team, create a new sculpture or pray deeply with a particular image of God before us, we are modifying and adjusting the interaction between what is happening at the interface of our neurons and our perceiving mind, which cannot be limited simply to have solely arisen independently from our brain cells. The significance of this will become clear as we are drawn more deeply into the plot of the story shame wants to tell.

Although at first this working definition of the mind felt a bit over-whelming to Justin, he found relief in discovering that his experience was not merely some abstract phenomenon that took place "in his head." Rather, it had concrete connections within his physicality that he could begin to alter. And soon we turned our attention to one of the principal features of a mind that is thriving, something that shame targets in its bid to undermine God's intended creation of goodness and beauty.

## THE INTEGRATED MIND

Think of a business, one that comprises several departments. To flourish, this business requires each department to function effectively in its par-ticular sphere, having adequate resources for its assigned tasks, be that the executive team, sales, marketing, research and development, or human resources. However, each of these departments must also com-municate well with one another. How else will a marketing agent or sales-person know which product to offer? This is an example of the phe-nomenon of *integration*. An integrated system is one in which its subset parts reflect *differentiation* and *linkage*: each part is differentiating or maturing in a proper way while growing in its linkage or connection to the others. Similarly, the mind can be described as having multiple func-tional domains. In order for the mind to function well, each of these domains must grow and mature (differentiate) but must simultaneously be connected to (link) the other domains. The responsibility for main-taining this connection lies in the action of the prefrontal cortex—that part of the brain that makes us most uniquely human. When we pay attention to these different activities of the mind, we are better positioned to be aware of their changes and shifts, and so better regulate them, rather than having them be in control of us.

Daniel Siegel conceived the expression "interpersonal neurobiology" in his landmark work *The Developing Mind*. In his later work, *Mindsight*, he has described nine different domains or functions of the mind and how their integration contributes to robust mental health. Integration, therefore, refers to the growth and maturation of each domain in its ability to do what it is designed to do, while simultaneously linking with other domains. Thus they are in fluid communication with each other. As we explore each domain, be aware that these suggest our current knowledge of brain science. As this changes and grows in the future, we may consider these domains differently.

Briefly then, the nine domains of the mind as described by Siegel are as follows.[5]

*Consciousness. Consciousness* refers to our general level of awareness of what we are sensing, perceiving, feeling, thinking and doing at any given moment. Attention is the hallmark feature of this domain. How truly conscious we are depends on how well we are paying attention to what we pay attention to.

*Vertical.* Our brains develop from the bottom up; that is to say, our brain stem (responsible for our heart and respiratory rates, appetite, sleep–wake cycle, elements of sexual arousal, and our flight or fight response, to name a few) develops first, followed by our limbic circuitry (one particular area where a great deal of what we perceive as emotion emerges), followed by our neocortex (the part of the brain responsible for processing sensory input from within our body and the environment, making decisions, reflection, logical processing, concrete creativity, the capacity to employ restraint, and consideration of consequences for our actions, just to name a very few).

*Horizontal.* The brain also develops laterally as two halves, the right and left hemispheres, with the right's growth in connection of its neurons tending to outpace the left's in the first eighteen to twenty-four months of life, the left quickly beginning to catch up soon after. The two hemispheres tend to house particular functions, the right being the center of visuospatial orientation, nonverbal communication, an integrated internal map of the body, and emotion; the left tends to be the center for the development of much (though not all) of language as well as our logical, linear and literal thought processing. One way to think of this is that, over time, the left brain works to make sense of what the right brain is sending it.

*Memory.* Memory is, among other things, as much about anticipating the future as it is about recalling the past. We remember things in order to predict what our futures will be like: Where did I put my keys so I can find them when I need to leave? Is it safe to allow my feelings to be revealed, given my experience of sharing them in the past? Is God to be trusted? Our *implicit* memory first develops through various bodily sensations, feelings, perceptions and nonconsciously intended behaviors. But eventually *explicit* memory is activated as we begin to remember facts ($3 \times 2 = 6$) along with what we call autobiographical memory, or our ability to remember the emotional as well as factual details of past events in our lives, as well as anticipate a particular future.

*Narrative.* As our minds develop, eventually we try to make sense of our lives. We take the input from our awareness of our conscious, vertical, horizontal and memory domains, and begin to tell our stories, with most of that content being nonverbal and nonconscious in nature. This narrative is highly influenced by our most intimate attachment relationships. Thus, who I am (i.e., what I tell myself about myself in visual images, sensations and feelings as well as words) is always going to be understood in terms of my current relationships—and by *current* I am referring to all relationships, past or present, that currently are influencing my mind's activity. Thus, even people who are deceased can continue to have sway over my life, depending on how I continue to process my ongoing experiences with my memory of them. This is why I can continue to have feelings of shame when I have memories of events involving a parent who is no longer living.

*State.* The phrase *state of mind*, as it turns out, represents a real, embodied phenomenon. Neuroscientists think of mental states as being highly correlated with specific neural network activity. Hence, when I am getting ready to play tennis, the firing pattern of my brain's neurons is quite different from when I am having an argument with my spouse.

We transition from state to state throughout our day, often without recognizing it. When I leave work to go home, my mind transitions from one state to the other. The real question is whether I am paying attention to this shift and all of its implications (e.g., I am going where it will be easier to let down my guard and be less careful with my reactions than it is at my workplace). Much of what creates trouble for us in life is related to our unexpected movement from one state to another or our inattentiveness to that type of transition.

*Interpersonal.* For all that convinces me that my mind is limited to "me," the truth remains that a great deal of my mind's activity is wrapped up with thinking about or interacting with other people's minds. This points to what Siegel refers to as "the neurobiology of we." In other words, there is rarely anything I do that is not either influencing or being influenced by other minds. And shame has no trouble swimming in the current that is constantly flowing between us.

*Temporal.* As far as we know, humans are the only creatures who have the capacity to *reflect* on their past and their future. This is not the same as remembering where I put the acorns because I want to eat this winter. Rather, it refers to our ability to give meaning to the things we remember. As such, we are aware that we had a beginning and that we will die at some point in the future. This awareness of time and its passing has great influence on how we respond to the present moment.

*Transpirational.* Siegel coined *transpirational* to refer to the process of attending to the preceding eight domains simultaneously. The overall implication is that to be aware of the activity of one's mind is a matter of hard work. Liberating work, no doubt, but hard nonetheless. However, as we proceed through the rest of this book we will see that if we are not attending to them, shame will have a much easier time wreaking havoc on all of them.

To recap, then, the central nervous system progresses in its development from bottom to top and right to left, the tendency being for the parts of our embodied mind that are lower in function and sophistication (not necessarily in terms of importance) to develop initially, followed by the parts of the brain that make us most uniquely human. This

# THE HUMAN BRAIN

**Looking from the outside toward the lateral portion of the left side of the brain:**

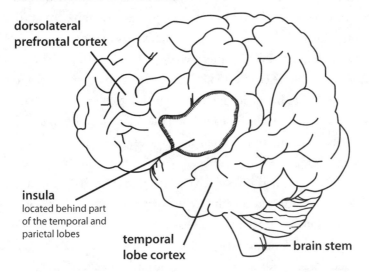

**dorsolateral prefrontal cortex**

**insula**
located behind part of the temporal and parietal lobes

**temporal lobe cortex**

**brain stem**

**Looking from the middle to the right side of the brain:**

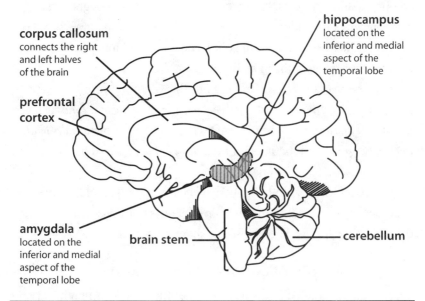

**corpus callosum**
connects the right and left halves of the brain

**prefrontal cortex**

**hippocampus**
located on the inferior and medial aspect of the temporal lobe

**amygdala**
located on the inferior and medial aspect of the temporal lobe

**brain stem**

**cerebellum**

**Figure 2.1. The human brain**

progression climaxes with the maturation of the prefrontal cortex (PFC) (see figure 2.1). At the level of the PFC those circuits emerging from "bottom to top" and "right to left" converge in order to communicate with each other. Over the course of the development of these nine domains we move from relatively lesser to greater degrees of complexity in our connections both intra- and interpersonally. As we age, our brains become more connected within themselves and mature in healthy ways as we also become more connected in healthy ways to other people. It is the task of the PFC to be the locale for integration to take place between these various domains. Cells here facilitate the differentiation of and the linkage between the different domains.

This way of comprehending the healthy development of the mind reminds us of the Genesis narrative which declares that we mysteriously hewn creatures are both dust and breath (Genesis 2:7); we are inseparably embodied and relational. Furthermore, this feature of integration is reflected in the psalmist's plea that God would give him an undivided heart (Psalm 86:11), and God's deep desire to do so while transforming hardened, disintegrated hearts into flexible, connected ones (Ezekiel 11:19). The notion that my mind comprises different parts that function well only when brought together in harmony *and only with assistance from someone outside of myself* is but one metaphor the writers of Scripture offer, a poetic expression of our embodied neural circuitry operating in an integrated fashion.

In the same manner that God intends that our minds grow in maturity and connection, just as we do with each other, *it is one of shame's primary features to disrupt and dis-integrate that very process, functionally leading to either rigid or chaotic states of mind and behavior, lived out intra- and interpersonally.*

It had become clear to Justin that every single domain of his mind had become disintegrated, not only over the course of the abuse he had endured but also in his response to his shame that emerged as a result.

### NEURONS THAT FIRE TOGETHER WIRE TOGETHER

Evidence accumulated in the last three decades indicates that brain cells have greater capacity for adaptation and regeneration than was previously believed. This characteristic is generally referred to as neuroplasticity. This property of neurons allows for the connection between different domains of the brain, and thereby different functional components such as sensations, images, feelings, thoughts and bodily actions. This is popularly recounted in what has become known as Hebb's axiom, in honor of Canadian neuropsychologist Donald Hebb: Those neurons that fire together wire together. In essence, the more we practice activating particular neural networks, the more easily they are to activate, and the more permanent they become in the brain.

In his epistle to the church in Rome, St. Paul suggests that renewal is possible:

> I urge you, brothers and sisters, in view of God's mercy, to offer your bodies as a living sacrifice, holy and pleasing to God—this is your true and proper worship. Do not conform to the pattern of this world, but be transformed by the renewing of your mind. Then you will be able to test and approve what God's will is—his good, pleasing and perfect will. (Romans 12:1-2)

It is fair to say that although Paul was not a neuroscientist, he refers here to what we now see through the lens of neuroplasticity. Renewal of the mind, therefore, is not just an abstraction. It means real change in real bodies.

As Justin told his story over several months, he began to make sense of how the very act of relational closeness activated associated neural networks of shame and fear that he had no explanation for. The fact that these networks were first formed when his brain was more neuroplastically malleable during his early adolescent years meant that they were more easily and permanently shaped. No wonder it was so difficult for him to alter this pattern, despite an Ivy League education and socioeconomic affluence at an early age.

Thus we see that the more we practice firing neurons in a particular way, the more easy it is to activate that particular pathway, and thus the more entrenched those patterns become, desirable or undesirable though they may be. We will turn again to neuroplasticity later in this book when considering the healing of shame.

## ATTENTION: THE IGNITION KEY OF THE MIND

*Neuroplasticity* is the feature of flexible adaptation that makes possible the connection (or pruning) of neural networks and thus the formation and permanence of shame patterns. And *attention* is the function that drives the movement of neuroplasticity. Via intentional attunement we connect the neurons located within the PFC with the neural networks correlated with the nine previously listed domains. By this attention we move them toward differentiation and linkage, bringing them together as an integrated whole. Attention is the engine of the mind's train that pulls along the rest of the functional cars. Ultimately we become what we pay attention to, and the options available to us at any time are myriad, the most important of which being located within us. Paul, in his letter to the Romans knows this, stating flatly, "Those who live according to the flesh have their minds set on what the flesh desires; but those who live in accordance with the Spirit have their minds set on what the Spirit desires. The mind governed by the flesh is death, but the mind governed by the Spirit is life and peace" (Romans 8:5-6). To have one's mind set on something is essentially about paying attention. What do I pay attention to? Paul says that what we pay attention to doubles back and governs us. Hence our attention is deeply associated with either death or life.

So much of the biblical narrative is the story of God working hard to get our attention. From Adam to Moses to Samuel to Isaiah to Jesus' disciples, from our church pulpit to our small group, from our kitchen to our bedroom to our boardroom, ours is a story of a people for whom paying attention—for whom keeping our mind on "whatever is true, whatever is noble, whatever is right, whatever is pure, whatever is lovely, whatever is admirable . . . excellent or praiseworthy" (Philippians 4:8)—is very hard work. As it is, most of what brings people into my office is a function of the degree to which they do not pay attention to much of what their mind is doing. Shame would have it no other way, and it routinely takes advantage of this tendency. When we do not attend in helpful ways to the various features our mind offers us, unfortunate things happen.

Take, for instance, when my wife asks, "Are you going to wear *that*?" Noticing the stung look on my face in response, she immediately follows with "I am just trying to be helpful." (*Excuse me? I think. Helpful? How in any universe is your commentary on the pants I am wearing "helpful"?*) If my PFC is not engaged and I am not paying attention to the sudden rise in my body's tension or the emotional sense of having been criticized or the thought, *She thinks I'm stupid when it comes to clothing*, which in about two nanoseconds leads to *She thinks I'm stupid, period*, I will soon be wishing to retract the words "Please, *don't* be helpful" that spew from my mouth. For in those four words, I, carried along by my facial expression, tone of voice and body language, launch a regional war that will leave us both feeling very hurt. Who knew that shame could exploit a pair of Dockers?

You would think that I could deflect such a small comment about my apparel, and that I would not take it so personally. How can such a small thing lead to an argument, the residue of which lasts the rest of the day? Here too we see the role of attention. Once shame begins its march from a small slight, growing to geometric expansion, my attentional mechanism goes offline and remains so. Reversing this shaming event is as much about getting my attention back on track as anything else. For Justin, the emotion of shame was so intense that it took him many weeks to begin to see changes in his capacity to direct his attention. But change he did. And we will see in future chapters how we go about doing that.

## THE PRIMACY OF EMOTION

One cannot speak about the mind without eventually wading into the amorphous world of emotion. I say "eventually" because when the word *mind* is mentioned, many if not most people first associate it with the process of how we think. However, when it comes to the development of the mind, we find that logical, linear thought processing is one of the last features to emerge. Indeed, emotion holds a place of primacy in the realm of human behavior. By *primacy* I am not implying that emotion is the most important of our mental functions, but rather that it tends to be primal, or early in the course of our mind's development. Responding to sensations, emotion is the mental activity that most fundamentally alerts us to transitions from state to state. And although researchers have not developed consensus on how to characterize it,[6] they do agree to emotion being the energy around which the brain organizes itself.[7]

When we examine human behavior we find that if we take emotion out of the equation, we stop moving. The derivation of the word *emotion* includes its Latin root, *a-motion*, which means "to precede movement." This suggests that whatever emotion is, it energizes and gives rise to human movement. From the time we are born, emotion is a primary driving force of our existence. If attention is the ignition key of the mind, then emotion is the fuel in the tank the engine runs on. Developmentally, emotion is present far earlier than cognition. Many researchers believe that it is present and active even before birth. Hence, emotion is of primal significance when it comes to our doing anything.

In order to talk about emotion we tend to separate it from other mental activity such as sensation, imagery or cognition. But in the mind there are no such distinct compartments. Although different regions of the brain are more dominantly correlated with particular mental activity, virtually everything that we experience is shaped and influenced by emotional tone. As such, emotion is something that both regulates us and that we regulate. Whenever we are thinking or sensing something, emotion is part of the process. It would therefore be more accurate to consider emotion as being woven throughout all human activity, albeit in degrees that are more or less perceptible to us in conscious ways. Therefore, there is never a time in which we are *not* "being emotional."

One particular way that emotions affect us is via our memory. We tend to attune to and thereby remember things that have emotional salience. Not that something need always be pleasant. Rather we attend to important and relevant things, and so practice remembering them. The more I practice remembering things I am emotionally drawn to, the more I become that which I remember.

When Justin described the things he would say to himself such as *That was so stupid!* it was not difficult to identify the words; he told me that he needed to "stop saying those things to myself." But underneath the words lay the feelings, and these were not as easy to identify or to stop. Consequently, he found that after some time of simply trying to forcibly stop himself from saying the words, the feelings still remained. He then reported, "Even though I'm not speaking the words, I still feel bad." The emotional quality of his experience continued, through practiced attention—even and especially unconscious practice—to fuel his repeated self-shaming behavior.

Another important aspect of emotional salience involves its role in our anticipation of the future. Indeed, when we imagine our future state, whether five minutes or five years from now, we are not merely thinking comprehensively about events, as such. The most salient feature that our brain anticipates is our emotional state. For example, if I am worried about what diagnosis the doctor will give to my child, I am not only worried about the *fact* that she may have cancer. Rather, my mind is anticipating what I will *feel* when I hear the news. Moreover, it is not only that I anticipate the feeling of deep sadness; even more important, *I anticipate being powerless to escape the feeling*. Awareness of this is crucial, for shame *as an emotion* is something we not only anticipate but also *feel* unable to change.

Of course, the reality is that at that future time of feeling sadness about my child's diagnosis, I will take some action that will mitigate it. The challenge is that emotion can so dominate my mind's landscape that it becomes difficult to extract myself from what I anticipate I will feel in the future and shift my attention to the present moment. The very act of attending to the present moment shifts my attention away from the overall experience of shame, but its power to prevent me from realigning my attention can indeed be quite overwhelming.

Emotion, then, courses throughout the entirety of our daily lives, giving rise to varying bandwidths of experience. We symbolize these different feelings with words such as *joy, sadness, anger, surprise, disappointment* and others, including *shame*. This implies that what is most primal and potent about shame is its emotional nature. It certainly can emerge in response to information provided for us, and therefore it seems to have its origin in cognition, but its power lies in our *felt* experience of it. It is important to keep this in mind, for when it comes to combating shame, if we are not attending to what we are feeling, it will be easy for it to have its way with us without our even knowing it.

## ATTACHMENT AND THE BRAIN

Attachment is the process that we each undergo, either relatively securely or insecurely, whereby as we are born we connect—attach—to important caregivers in our lives in response to their particular approach to us. This connection is first accomplished via skin-to-skin contact, through the sounds and tones of voices, eye contact, body language and eventually is solidified as a child comes to comprehend language-based communication.

Technically, *attachment* refers to the process by which the immature infant brain accesses and utilizes the strengths of the mature adult brain in order to learn how to organize and regulate itself. Our first means of learning how to regulate our attention, memory, emotion and many other functions of the mind depends on another brain, and to some degree this continues for our entire lives. Over the course of our lives the relative health of our attachment has far-reaching implications for our flourishing, and strongly influences the eventual nature and health of the relationships we develop and maintain into adulthood. It shapes the way we interact with others, what kind of friendships and marriages we will have, and then reinforces the cycle by influencing how we parent our own children.

Every newborn comes into the world looking for someone looking for her. When a baby is born, she enters the world with a particular temperament, eliciting a response from her parents, hopefully one that will be properly attuned to her needs. But their approach to her will be deeply shaped not only—and not even mostly—by their new baby's temperament, but also, and dominantly, by their own developmental story that has shaped how they navigate relationships, how well they have learned to sense and regulate their own emotion, how they notice and respond to the emotional cues of others (especially the nonverbal ones), and to what degree they have made coherent sense of their own story with all of its beauty and brokenness. Depending on how her parents approach her, the baby will attach in a relatively secure or in-secure fashion. To the degree that parents have done the necessary work to develop their own integrated minds, they will be able to foster secure attachment in their child. As Siegel has said, of all the variables that encourage the development of secure attachment in a child, the single most powerful one is the degree to which the child's parent has made coherent sense of his or her own story.[8]

Secure attachment is fostered in environments in which there is a premium placed on empathy, attunement, mindfulness and the proper setting of limits—features that had not always been present in Justin's childhood home. Rather, perfectionism, not only of how he performed in school but also what he believed theologically, was elevated above all other virtues. Justin even perceived following Jesus to be something that needed to be done perfectly, albeit without those words ever being spoken directly. It was more in the way he interpreted all the nonverbal cues that led to his assumptions about never revealing imperfections— and certainly never ones that involved sexuality.

It is noteworthy that secure attachment is also highly correlated with the maturation of several functions of the prefrontal cortex, including body regulation, attuned communication, emotional balance, fear modulation, response flexibility, empathy, insight and intuition. This reinforces the notion that the nature of relationships contingently affects the wiring of neuronal connections in our brains, something that is taking place at all times. This reflects, again, an anthropology that asserts that we were created fundamentally as connected beings, mirroring a communal God who, as the writer of Genesis 1:26 portrays, wants to create humankind to be "in *our* likeness." Not like "me" or simply like nothing else that had been created. Rather, from the beginning the triune God made us in such a way so that we could join the three divine persons in their circle of creativity. Creativity of which one hallmark is joy. The natural progression, then, of the development of integrated minds, relationships and communities is fully realized in the experience of joy—joy even in the presence of very hard places. For secure attachment is not primarily about the absence of pain but the presence of joy in the face of those challenging places. It is not about the absence of ruptures but the faithful repair of ruptures, even when repair seems beyond the reach of our imaginations. Shame of course will do everything it can to interfere with the emergence of joy, curiosity and the creativity that inevitably ensues—even in the face of difficult relational circumstances.

Not surprisingly, therefore, our patterns of attachment deeply influence the way we experience our relationship with God. For he has to deal with the same brain that we do; he engages the same proclivities we have for avoiding or being anxious about the intimacy of relationships. It is not as if we get to put our brains, which are wired in a particular way through our attachment patterns, on the shelf and somehow draw on a separate one when it comes to dealing with God. He comes to the same set of neural networks that our friends, parents, spouse, children or enemies do.

In Genesis 2:18 God says, "It is not good for the man to be alone. I will make a helper suitable for him." The idea of being alone, or in this case, "incomplete," was something that God cared about and remedied by making and bringing a woman to the man (Genesis 2:22). This text also, however, is a harbinger of what is to come later in the story, suggesting that the dark side of being alone—really alone: isolated, deserted, forgotten, dismissed, scorned, pushed out, abandoned—is a potential that God recognized. And we will soon see how shame is deeply committed to exploiting the machinery of attachment in creating states of aloneness within us and between us, and most substantially between us and God. But just as this mind–brain–relational triad can be disintegrated by shame, so also are relationships, through earned secure attachment (an echo of God coming to us embodied in Jesus), the means by which shame is regulated and healed.

## KEEPING STORYTELLING IN MIND

One of the important features of the mind that emerges from our attachment processes is not just *that* but *how* we tell stories. As the complex matrix of our neuro-relationships matures together, grounded in our attachment patterns, it becomes the soil out of which grows the first shoots of our storytelling tendencies. This had become true for Justin, as it is true for each of us.

What starts as a "simple" set of responses to nonverbal cues that has me firmly, albeit securely or insecurely, attached to my caregivers by as early as seven months eventually matriculates into what I tell myself, silently or out loud, in words, images and feelings about everything I believe about myself and the universe: *I'm so glad my dad loves me. She will never amount to anything. I love Dave Matthews's music. I can't stop drinking. She's a great teacher. Those immigrants are going to ruin the country. Jesus loves me. God must be so disappointed in me. I love my work as an engineer. She doesn't care about my feelings. I'm so grateful to be forgiven. I'm not pretty enough. I love my marriage. I'm afraid I'll never be married. I love sex. I hate sex. Why am I so stupid? That joke was hilarious!* The list is endless.

We are storytellers. We yearn to tell and hear stories of goodness and beauty, and this is the echo of God's intention. We long for our stories to be about joy, not just reflections of what we believe but of who we *are*, who we long to *be*. But recall that so much of the mind's activity, and our way of telling stories, is done beneath the radar of consciousness, let alone language, immersed in sensations, images and feelings along with thoughts.[9] But shame wants very much to infect every element of the mind in order to distort God's story and offer another narrative.

We now turn to explore the explicit nature of how shame operates within and between our minds, fulfilling its role as evil's vector of disintegration of the creation. In so doing, we will first be introduced to the hallmark of God's creative purpose, which marks us as people who "have a hope and a future," albeit not one we easily remember.

## 3

# Joy, Shame and the Brain

Jackie was born into a world of poverty that eventually led to home-lessness. Her mother had done the best she could, but Jackie found herself moving from one foster care home to another. Her mother was unable to care for her physical needs, and her father was out of the picture.

Every element of her life shouted shame at her: her embarrassment in elementary school when she was unable to invite friends to her home because of its disarray; her self-consciousness about her clothing, which was worn and often unkempt; the sympathetic glances of teachers and social workers that felt more patronizing than kind; the foster families that repeatedly sent her elsewhere, giving the clear message that Jackie was unwanted. Almost every aspect of her young life was marked by shame.

But life takes funny turns. During her freshman year at one of the local high schools, Jackie had a chance encounter with some girls who had less interest in appearances and more interest in Jesus and real relationships. They invited her to a Young Life meeting where she was introduced to the leader, Kerry, who took her under her wing. But Jackie's was not a linear story that moved ceaselessly in a positive direction. Shame was not about to go quietly into the night. Over the next four years life took turns at times hopeful, at others painful. Between the drugs and the sex and the mean boyfriends, Jackie's Young Life leader remained. And prayed. And remained. And eventually Jackie, depressed and discouraged, found her way into my office, and then to a group for adolescent girls that taught her what it means to be known, to be understood, to be loved. She had been depressed enough that we decided an anti-depressant was in order, which proved to be helpful.

We met with her biological mother as well as her current foster parents, a couple that was willing to stay the course. Jackie was bright and wanted to attend college, but the weight of all of her experience told her she did not have what it took, that life eventually would overtake her and plough her under. A constant voice reminded her that no matter what Kerry told her or lived before her, no matter how much medicine she took, no matter how much she went to church or to group therapy, she simply could not push back against the inertia of her life. This is shame on full display, in all of its awful narrating self.

And to be sure, many stories of brokenness do not turn directly into the light. But enough success in the classroom (with the help of a particular English teacher who saw in Jackie a gift for thoughtful, critical thinking and writing), along with what in hindsight seemed like a sea of relational capital invested in her life, landed Jackie a scholarship to a small liberal arts college. And in that community she found a campus ministry group, and in that campus ministry group she found Josh. And he found her. And in Josh's family she found depth and connection that was at first as unsettling as it was healing. Unsettling because she initially found herself waiting for the other shoe to drop, expecting Josh and his family to disappear, as had her home, parents and so many other relationships. As she would later tell me, "You know, if something seems too good to be true, it usually is."

So Jackie and Josh were married, and from that union baby Grace made her way into the world. When Grace was born, her parents were overwhelmed with feelings they could hardly put into words, especially Jackie. And with Grace's birth, joy was the signature emotion that announced to the world that goodness and beauty can prevail in the face of overwhelming shame.

This story provides a window through which we can begin to see what our lives are intended to be, how shame can so callously interrupt them, and the interpersonal neurobiological correlates for these occasions. What then goes on in the developing human mind that shame so intentionally targets and so powerfully disrupts? In what apparent interpersonal neurobiological direction are we naturally headed as we enter the world and from which shame so easily throws us off course? What should a fully integrated mind expect from the story it inhabits?

## WHAT IS THE CHIEF END OF MAN?

In 1892, writing in his diary, Leo Tolstoy wrote, "Life cannot have any other purpose than joy and goodness. Only this purpose—joy—is ultimately worthy of life."[1] This was long before the age of neuroscience, but long after the development of the Westminster Shorter Catechism, which in 1647 declared that the chief end of humankind is "to glorify God and enjoy him forever." Later C. S. Lewis, in his sermon titled "The Weight of Glory," writes of how "glory" for humans is hearing that we are pleasing to the One whose pleasure we most long to fulfill. It is no more realized than when we hear our Master say, "Well done!"[2] The common theme these voices herald is *joy*. They assume that the delight of God in trinitarian fellowship is nothing if not an invitational that he longs for us to join. The defining relational motif for humankind is not that we need to work as hard as we can, or at least harder than we are. It is not to do our best or to guarantee that our children will have a better life than we had. It is not about being right or the acquisition of power. Each of those (and other visions like them) play into the hand of shame's anxiety.

No—rather, we were created for joy. Not a weak and watery concept of joy that merely dilutes our sadness and pain. Rather it is the hard deck on which all of life finds its legs, a byproduct of deeply connected relationships in which each member is consummately known. But looking around at the world, it is not always easy to believe this. Jackie's first two decades on the planet certainly knew very little of this. Instead she mostly knew and learned how to survive something that felt repeatedly disintegrating and disorienting, leaving her with little in the way of coping tactics to correct her course. Her mind found few ways in which the intention for integration was realized—apart from the relational CPR she began to receive as an adolescent. Her story's early pages were largely written in the language of shame. Given so many disadvantages, how could she expect her mind and life to emerge into a state of joy? In a world where so much of God's story has been pushed to the margin of cultural belief, is it possible to find the life that the Gospels declare is true in the resurrection?

Fortunately, as the followers of Jesus assert (Acts 14:17), God does not leave himself without a witness. And one of those witnesses is his material creation. Here we see that not only our chief *end* but also our *beginning* is the vision of God's delight.

## Joy and the Integrated Mind

In the last twenty years, research spearheaded by the work of psychologist Allan Schore and others persuasively suggests that of all the primary tasks of the infant, there is none more crucial than the pursuit, acquisition and establishment of joyful, securely attached relationships.[3] This is not the place to explore the history of developmental psychology, but suffice to say that there has been much gained with Schore's work because it uses the horsepower of the data acquired from attachment research to educate us about the role of joy in the formation of an integrated mind.

The recent work of Jim Wilder and colleagues highlights the place of joy in our development across the life cycle, and its role as a relationally supported state that leads to human flourishing.[4] Wilder and his team drink deeply from the well of attachment research and the efforts of Schore in particular. But they go one step—many steps, in fact—further in translating Schore's work in terms of God's intention for our lives, from infancy to adulthood.

As Schore points out, joyful relationships develop as parents attune properly to the needs of the infant in such a way that it fosters secure attachment. One of the fundamental aspects of secure attachment is the infant's enlarging sense of the presence of a "secure relational base" from which he or she can explore the world. As is the case for any system, whether a human cell or a nation, without the presence of safety, little to no creative activity can ensue.

Thus, when babies feel emotionally safe (which necessarily presumes physical safety), they are free to engage their surrounding environment, learning not only about the world but their responses to it. They grow in their joy of curiosity and discovery. Even when they encounter danger or noxious stimuli (e.g., falling and scraping a knee; trying to eat begonias) or sustain a rupture in relationship (e.g., crossing a limit appropriately set by a parent, subsequently having to endure the negative consequences of that choice), a secure attachment provides for the healing and repair of that distress or rupture. In this way even in the face of temporarily unpleasant affect, babies' sense of curiosity and grounding in joy are preserved. As we explored in chapter two however, this depends most significantly on the states of mind of the parents.

Joy then can be understood as *the* primary positive developmental affect in whose presence the process is grounded. We recall that integration is a *contingent* process, one in which the mind of the child is working interdependently and in response to the *intentions* of the adult, a process out of which joy emerges. This joy circles back to reinforce the positive anticipation of further interaction between the parent and child. It is also noteworthy that this affective response of joy is not solely isolated within the child's mind, but is shared. It is not simply joy for joy's sake but rather that joy is the signature indication of deep, mindful, intentional connection. It is contingent on an interpersonal process in which the infant essentially hears from the parent, among other things, "I am so glad to be with you!" The work of Carol Dweck points to another rendition of this in the anticipated voice of "Well done!" in the wake of having worked hard at a task, *even if the goal you wanted to reach has not been realized.*[5] And who doesn't want to continue to hear that throughout his or her lifetime?

As children age the nature of their curiosity, exploration and creativity naturally becomes more complex. To the degree that joy precedes and follows this growth, established in the matrix of secure attachment, integration of the highest order ensues. Children move from playroom to classroom to construction site or restaurant kitchen to economics to forestry to mothering or fathering to welding to vacationing to . . . you name it. In this way, a secure base, no matter how old a "child" is, creates the context for exploration, proper risk and extension into realms of imagined experience that is, as the Victorian poet Robert Browning hints in *Andrea del Sarto*, beyond the child's and then the adult's grasp.[6]

Joy, then, becomes a prominent affect around which the integration process gravitates. In chapter two we learned of the importance of integration and the nine domains of the mind that Siegel refers to. These domains most fully come to a place of differentiation and linkage in the context of joyful interpersonal connection.

There is no domain that the creative power of joy, given the right nutrients in the soil, cannot grow in. It is to the world's advantage that the parent, teacher, coach, pastor, police officer, emergency room nurse, middle manager, CEO, boat captain and farmer cultivate cultures of joy. Jackie seldom experienced these cultures before her high school years. This is important as we wade into the neuroscience of shame, for shame most primitively and powerfully undermines the process of joyful attachment, integration and creativity.

## EARLY OUT OF THE GATE

What then is the interpersonal neurobiological nature of shame? We have just explored the notion and nature of joy in order to provide the necessary contrast against shame's disintegrating forces.

It is crucial to note from the outset that *shame* as a neurophysiologic phenomenon is not bad in and of itself. It is, rather, our system's way of warning of possible impending abandonment, although we do not think of it in those terms, and certainly not at very early ages. However, our problem with it is generally that we tend to respond to it by relationally moving away from others rather than toward them, while experiencing within our own minds a similar phenomenon of internal disintegration. Moreover, our response is largely a function of how we collaborate—or don't—with the relational capital we share with others that, when accessed appropriately, will lead to growth and connection.

Shame makes its way into our stories at an early age. So early, in fact, that we usually have no conscious memory of our initial encounters with it. This can take place as early as fifteen to eighteen months, and usually involves a child's response to someone's nonverbal cues—a glance, tone of voice, body language, gestures or intensity of behavior—that interrupt whatever the child may be doing, delivering a subtle but undeniably felt message of disapproval.[7] This is something that initially *is translated as something sensed and a child responds to primarily as a function of the body.* It is not something a child first responds to by *thinking rationally with words*, for often his or her brain is not yet so well-developed to comprehend them. Rather a response will be generated largely from neurons in the child's right hemisphere, where so much of his or her world is being lived in the first eighteen to twenty-four months of life.

(As an aside, this early development in part reflects how we differentiate between the emotional states of shame and guilt. Researchers have described *shame* as a feeling that is deeply associated with a person's sense of self, apart from any interactions with others; *guilt,* on the other hand, emerges as a result of something I have done that negatively affects someone else. Guilt is something I feel because I have *done* something bad. Shame is something I feel because I *am* bad. In fact, when in its grip, it is quite difficult for us to separate our self from the shame that we are feeling. Guilt, on the other hand, only emerges when a child's brain is mature enough [around three to six years] to be aware that his or her behavior negatively affects the emotional state of another. Furthermore, a necessary element of the emotion we call guilt includes empathy, if even in primitive form. In order for me to feel guilt, I must in some way simultaneously feel the pain I have caused for another. In this sense guilt tends to draw my attention to another and is often accompanied by a desire to resolve the problem by being closer to him or her [admitting a wrongdoing, seeking and being offered forgiveness]. Shame, on the other hand, separates me from others, as my awareness of what I feel is virtually consumed with my own internal sensations. Furthermore, they are related in that I will sense shame in addition to the guilt I feel when I do something "wrong." Hence, in one sense, neurodevelopmentally guilt stands on shame's shoulders. One way to think of this is that we can experience shame without guilt but are unlikely to experience guilt without shame.)[8]

Furthermore, from a brain standpoint, the interchange between adult and child that shame exploits is dependent on the regulatory balance between the child's sympathetic and parasympathetic nervous systems. These two systems, both of which derive from the brainstem, unconsciously and involuntarily influence the emotional tone of the mind in an ongoing fashion.[9] The sympathetic system is correlated with arousal and is activated when a person is engaged in something that has a positively anticipated outcome, whether movement toward a relational connection or a creative activity such as play or work, or as Siegel describes it, it behaves like the gas pedal of a car's engine, providing fuel of emotional energy.[10] The parasympathetic system is correlated with the slowing of a person's behavior, acting more like a brake. Under normal developmental circumstances the emotional tone set by these systems is regulated by the prefrontal cortex, acting as a neurobiological clutch, keeping a balance between arousal and diminution of the mind's energy. For each of us, our PFC has to learn to do its work as a clutch; our connection to adult caretakers provides the classroom for this type of learning.

When a toddler is first being introduced to limits and hears Mom say "No!" she is activating the child's parasympathetic system, helping it apply the brake to his or her sympathetic system's engagement with running toward the stairs or, for that matter, engaging in any behavior that is legitimately unacceptable, impulsive or potentially relationally threatening. In these cases, shame is to be equated with the emerging neurophysiologic response that every child must integrate in order to develop self-regulatory capacity. When Mom says "No!" the toddler does not necessarily understand the literal, abstract meaning of *no*—the brain is not yet well-developed enough for this. The child responds mostly to the tone of her voice, given that at this point a toddler's right hemisphere is still largely running the mind's show. The child is simply doing what his or her brain wants to do, blissfully unaware of any danger. Upon hearing Mom's voice, he or she may feel a sudden, minor discomfort accompanied by feeling startled, along with blushing. In these moments, when the parent is attuned to the child's emotional responses, "no" is delivered in an attuned manner, even in what seems to be a somewhat urgent situation, with nonverbal cues that balance the message with firmness while maintaining relational connection. Hearing the sharpness in her voice, which interrupts the child's movement, he or she next hears it soften as Mom says, "Let's go this way!" quickly moving physically to redirect the child elsewhere. Joy is not at risk of being undermined, even in the instance of limit-setting, when a parent's mind is attuned to maintaining connection with the child.

## THE SHEARING EFFECT OF SHAME

When shame strikes, however, the interchange is wholly different. It often occurs when we are moving in a direction of creative exploration, minding our own business, when an unexpected force of nature enters and brutally throws us off course. Crucial in this drama is our state of mind, which typically is one of unsuspecting, trusting anticipation as we venture forward in some endeavor. We are simply doing what we joyfully—or at the very least unconcernedly—intend to be doing, such as coloring or running through the house or throwing a baseball near windows or asking for a new bike or writing a report for the supervisor or entering a romantic relationship or taking a risk investing money or choosing to believe in Jesus. Creative adventure has no age limits.

Or in Jackie's case, when she hopefully asked her mother if she could invite some of her classmates over to her house to play. Suddenly, out of the blue comes the *unexpected shearing effect* of shame. When her mother answers irritably, "No! How many times have I told you we can't do that?" there is a certain shearing off of joyful anticipation, a blindsiding that overtakes her and completely catches her off-guard. There is no clutch involved in the application of the brake of the parasympathetic system to the sympathetic system's energy, no gradual or mindful engagement while attempting to change the direction of her intended course (asking for friends to come to her house). Her arousal is precipitously unhinged, like so many colliding railway cars piling up behind the mind's engine as it has come to a screeching halt.

With this truncation of a person's creative movement, there ensues for her a series of physiologic events, including a lowering and turning away of her gaze, a heaviness in her chest, an uncomfortable fullness in her head, a wave of an intensified blushing effect that courses over her entire body, and a turning in toward herself and away from others.[11] In terms of mental processes, the distinct feeling of shame, one we all know but sometimes find hard to put into words, quickly arises. A deep sense of self-consciousness emerges; cognition becomes fuzzy as our thoughts are disabled; words may be hard to find (if we are old enough to form them); and the mind becomes caught in a vortex of images, sensations and thoughts that recycle and feed on each other at light speed, reinforcing the experience. It becomes difficult to imagine a way to halt the internal state of affairs, feeling trapped in a mind-body maze of emotional nausea. Usually, this state will persist until we are able to extricate ourselves from the situation, the circumstance passes or someone acts in such a way to intervene on our behalf.

Furthermore, in a shame encounter that takes place before language is fully developed, it is not as if the child thinks in terms of *Mom isn't happy with me*—cognition is not yet developed enough for this. Rather, the child is being governed by the parts of the brain (brainstem, limbic circuitry and portions of the right hemisphere) that simply respond to emotional shifts. We first develop a felt sense of shame rather than a rational explanation of a series of events. With repeated exposure to events such as these, we pay attention to and, via our early neuroplastic flexibility, more permanently encode these shame networks. Thus, they become more easily able to fire later on, even when activated by the most minor or even unrelated stimuli.

## Shame's Disintegrating Effect

In response to this traumatic, shearing interaction with another person, the signature feature of shame is set in motion. When an individual, relationship or community is touched by it, the mind moves toward a more disintegrated state. Sensations, images, feelings, thoughts and behaviors have a more difficult time flowing as a coherent whole. The PFC cannot easily bring together the various functions of the mind, which are kept separated by the dividing energy of shame. In the same way that a destructive weather system (e.g., tornado, hurricane or flood) disrupts the connected infrastructure of power supply and people, so shame does to the mind and relationships.

With the introduction of the affect of shame, not only is each of Siegel's nine domains disrupted in its capacity to function well, but also the whole group of domains find it difficult to be connected. For instance, when I experience shame, I find it virtually impossible to turn my attention to something other than what I am feeling. I can become overwhelmed with the activity of my brainstem (the no-clutch phenomenon), and my PFC goes offline. I am not able to think coherently, and my logical thought processes, which usually help me make good choices, are unavailable to regulate my right brain, from which all of the emotion is pouring.

Furthermore, my memory is inundated with old, implicit network activity, recollections of other times I have felt this, and I am unable to marshal the necessary memories of strength and confidence I desperately need at the moment. Shame is overtaking me. I then begin to construct a narrative that predicts a bleak and pessimistic future. I am unable to tell the whole story, certainly not one in which I am loved by God unconditionally and life, in the end, will be okay. My state of mind is fully disrupted, and transitioning back to one of coherence and peacefulness requires enormous effort. I can only see myself as being intolerable to others, and I sense the impossibility that this feeling will ever end.

The process of disintegration therefore follows a predictable, inevitable trajectory, one that begins with separation and ends in the hell of utter isolation. It begins with physically turning away, which takes place upon shame's activation. In the same way that we turn our gaze down and away, so as to not see anyone seeing us, so also different functional parts of the mind turn away, so to speak, and are disintegrated from other functional parts. Our thinking and feeling and sensing turn away from each other, are disconnected from each other and from the centering, regulating care of the PFC. With shame, we involuntarily move out of the sight and the mind of other people as the sensations, images, feelings and thoughts of our own mind move out of the sightline and awareness of each other. Certainly with minor incidents we sense little in the way of disintegration. But with overly toxic events, it can feel as if we are literally going out of our minds.

This movement toward virtual infinite separation is our desperate attempt to deescalate the awful emotional sensation that we are enduring at the moment. For instance, in turning our gaze and body away from someone, we seek as expeditiously as possible to reduce the acutely painful feeling of being exposed. We are not aware that we simultaneously reinforce the deeply felt notion, captured via implicit memory tracts, that we are in fact shameful. Little do we know that this neuropsychological response in the long run only serves to reinforce our proclivity to reactivate the very state we are seeking to escape, not least because we often find ourselves having to cope with this state *by ourselves in isolation*—a state that decreases the flexibility and resilience of the mind—the very isolation that shame has created in the first place.

With disintegration and isolation comes another feature of shame that we don't at first recognize. When shame appears, especially in malignant forms, we are often driven to a felt sense of *stasis*. Our mind feels incapable of thinking. We may feel literally physically frozen in place when experiencing extreme humiliation, and if we are able to move, we feel like going somewhere we can hide and remain hidden without returning to engage others. We don't necessarily experience this with minor insults, but there is no question that our ability to move creatively in our mind is slowed. This general idea that shame leads the world ultimately to a point of paralysis, vis-à-vis the movement that is required for creative engagement, will become more important when we explore the nature of God's movement and its necessity for shame's healing.

What begins in the mind as the separation of its various functions, and leads to the isolation of each from the other, is eventually expressed in the world of relationships—from family to friendships to communities to nations—leaving them fractured and impotent to regain any sense of relational integrity. This is shame at its worst. No one needs to believe in God to know that this is the way it works. We have all been there and know this experience of disintegration to be true. The question, of course, is what to do when this storm front blows into our living room.

## Mostly About Me, but Not Only About Me

A disintegrating outbreak of shame deeply affects one's sense of self. However, although we experience our shame response emerging wholly and independently within us, it does so *in response to an encounter we have with someone else.* Its very nature is such that on reflection, we not only feel shame, we feel responsible for the feeling, a shaming experience in and of itself, which is again a reflection of shame's tendency to be self-referential. I not only *feel* bad, I have the sense that I *am* bad, independent of any role played by someone outside of me. However, it is important to note (especially later as we explore the world of storytelling) that no one ever feels the sharp sting of shame apart from an initial encounter with someone else that, despite perhaps even having no conscious intention to do so, activates the shame response. Hence, despite shame being *mostly* about me, it is never *only* about me, even when my experience of it seems to emerge fully and only from deep within the dungeon of my own mind.

At its worst, the sensation and emotional tone of shame is like none other. Few emotional states can match it for how unbearably painful it can be. We have learned that before it is something we know logically, as in "I feel ashamed because I behaved badly . . . I did not do well enough on my test . . . I am not good enough for my parents," we first become familiar with it at a lower brain-function level. However, eventually, as we do with any emotional experience we pay attention to, we begin to try to make sense of what we feel. We try to understand it using words and concepts. One word (certainly not the only or necessarily the best) that is deeply associated with the feeling of shame is *accused.* It is no wonder, given that despite our sense of shame being within us, we often endure it as something that has been foisted on us by virtue of the accusation of someone else. The notion of being accused, in its most malignant form, leads to a state symbolized by another word: *contempt.* This word represents deep derision and condescension. The research data on marriage offered by John Gottman is replete with evidence that one of the most powerful predictors of the likelihood that a marriage will not survive is the presence of contempt displayed by one partner toward another.[12] As we will see in chapter five, there is deep connection between what the Hebrew language refers to as "the Satan" as accuser and the notion of shame. For though we eventually carry the burden of shame by ourselves, we must never forget that there will always be someone outside my experience playing a collaborative role in the disintegration of my mind.

This notion of there being another involved in the dance of shame highlights the natural outflow of having been accused: judgment. I am not speaking of the word as it applies to wise discernment. Rather, to a posture of criticism and condescension that so easily and stealthily winds its way around our minds in response to our having felt accused. With little to no awareness, we seamlessly respond to shame with judgment, which emerges as words. But more significantly, these words carry the emotional arrows slung as much at ourselves as they are at others.

## DEATH OF A THOUSAND SHAMEFUL CUTS

This basic neurophysiologic pattern is played out in large and small ways incessantly in the course of our day-to-day lives. It is not that difficult to imagine its manifestation in Jackie's story, for hers is one in which shame showed up early and often in patently obvious ways. But for some if not many of us, and for much of our lives, shame is far subtler and easily hides in the shadows of what we assume to be normal life. Normal in that it involves interactions played out largely on the plane of nonconsciousness, interactions so common so as to be barely noticeable. As parents (or teachers, spiritual leaders, employers, artists or anyone else in positions of relational influence), we are often oblivious to much of our own intentional behaviors. These behaviors often unfold in micro-moments, as it were, of unconsciously derived nonverbal and verbal— yet intentional—acts. Though barely noticeable, we co-create schemas of shame that necessarily are woven into the fabric of the story that another tells about his or her life. Even in relatively healthy environments, let alone those of Jackie's story, shame shows up in ways that we might not first identify. Ethan eventually came to discover how his life reflected this.

Born into a family that loved God and each other, he was the third of five children. He recalled his to be "a really good Christian home." But for some reason Ethan was plagued with self-doubt and criticism. From the outside this was difficult to reconcile given his affable nature and his capacity for living effectively in his relational and work life. In fact, no small part of his complaint to me was that he felt like there was something wrong with him for having the experiences of self-judgment in the first place. He had no clear idea where that could be coming from. Given his life, how could he possibly have these thoughts and feelings?

However, it did not take long to discover that life in his family of origin was not unidimensional in its approach to emotion. It was not egregiously dysfunctional, but imperfect nonetheless. Ethan's father, who had grown up as the son of an angry alcoholic, while affectionate with his children, on occasion was sarcastic or condescending, or displayed impatience when they made mistakes or were unable to perform tasks around the home as well or as quickly as he expected. And there were the brief vents of irritation that would catch everyone off-guard. Ethan's mother tended to cover these episodes with comments such as, "Your dad has had a hard day" or "Don't let that bother you; you know he loves you." The problem was not just that these instances occurred (usually unpredictably) but that Ethan's father rarely if ever apologized for his behavior.

Hence, Ethan did not understand his story as one in which he had sustained terrible abuse. Rather, it illustrates how our experience of shame can form along a range of emotional states (from subtle and silent to grossly large and loud). For example, as Ethan knew, whenever he heard his father sigh when he was impatient with Ethan's help, the message was clear: Ethan was not enough. Not fast enough, smart enough, experienced enough. Just not enough. These words were never spoken; rather, it was the undertone of the nonverbal communication that carried the weight of the message. Again, we see that no matter how minor or overwhelming in its forcefulness, for Ethan, much like Jackie, shame is primarily sensed and felt as a shift in emotional tone. For all of us it often occurs in situations when we are moving in a direction of creative exploration, minding our own business, and into that exploratory space enters the wind shear of shame.

Thus, although much of his life was immersed in a milieu in which Jesus was honored, there were enough of these painful experiences— albeit comparatively insignificant relative to much of the world—that Ethan's inner life was frequently punctured with feelings of uneasiness and caution, and self-critical, pessimistic thoughts when confronted with the prospect of taking actions that required relational or vocational risk. Furthermore, he believed that he should not be having these responses in the first place because there was no overwhelming reason for them. He had never been raped or endured poverty; why on earth should he be bothered by this kind of trouble? Ethan's story illustrates how common it is for shame to be silently lodged and active in every nook and cranny of our lives when we have little to no idea of its presence. Which is exactly the way it wants things to be. There is no better place for shame to hide than in those stories in which it does not seem to be that prevalent.

## HARBINGER OF ABANDONMENT

As we discussed in chapter two, the mind flourishes when in relationships of intentionally attuned connection. As it turns out, humans tend to experience no greater distress than when in relationships of intentional, unqualified abandonment—abandoned physically and left out of the mind of the other. With shame, I not only sense that something is deeply wrong with me, but accompanying this is the naturally extended consequence that because of this profound flaw, you will eventually want nothing to do with me and will leave. Paradoxically, then, shame is a leveraging affect that anticipates abandonment while simultaneously initiating movement away—leaving. And we can leave in a hundred ways, some of them unknown to us, as Miriam found to be the case.

Smart and ambitious, Miriam had systematically been promoted in her work in the US government. She eventually landed a plum job that maximized her talents. But not long into her position she became aware that her supervisor, a well-respected policy developer, rarely spoke with her about his expectations for her work. Then, on unexpected occasions, he would call her into his office and critique her performance. Though he did not say it directly, she sensed what she interpreted to be his disappointment. This, of course, was bewildering to her. Her initial response to his criticism was to do what she had always done when her mistakes were revealed: work harder.

This pattern continued for six months. Despite agreeing with her to be more forthcoming with his expectations, his behavior changed very little. Within that span Miriam's confidence waned and her demeanor at the office became, not surprisingly, more subdued. She had always worked for employers who had treated her with respect and had drawn out the best in her. Even when pointing out places for improvement, people had been direct and kind. She had no category for understanding her current experience. By the time she came to see me, she was acutely depressed. Panic was overtaking her, she couldn't sleep and was unable to concentrate at work, which only made her circumstances more dire.

Her friends suggested her problem was her boss; furthermore, given her maturity and intelligence, they did not understand why she did not immediately see this as clearly as they did. Miriam, however, was having a hard time reconciling this. She had always done well—what was she doing wrong now? Her boss was so well-respected in the policy world, how could this be his fault? Certainly, given his success, this couldn't be his fault. Yes, she could possibly understand how his behavior might be contributing to her troubles, but it felt overwhelming to consider the implications that her condition might have everything to do with how he was treating her. What did that say about how she reads people? How did she not pick up on this when she interviewed with him for the position? What would she do if she quit this job? How could she get a favorable recommendation for another position?

She was part of a faith community and met regularly with a small group for prayer and reflection on Scripture. However, when she spoke of her situation, there was no small amount of embarrassment. This reality, that she was ashamed to report her experience to those who ostensibly would be empathic and supportive, was not lost on her. I inquired why this was so. How was it that a gospel that spoke of God's faithfulness and mercy, embodied as it was in this loving community, seemed to evoke the very opposite from within her?

She began to get a better handle on the situation when we started to explore her early developmental years. She recalled a close, open relationship with her mother. Though not perfect, she could be honest with her mother, even about her mother's faults. Her father, a successful businessman, though never unkind to her or anyone in her family, had always been emotionally reserved and distant. A good provider, he did not lavish words or gestures of affection and affirmation on the members of his family. When I asked Miriam to describe her relationship with him she replied, "Dad is the one person I can always count on. I know he loves me." I then asked how she knew that he loved her. She listed the things he routinely did for the family in terms of provision. When I asked what they actually talked about and the words he used to communicate his interest in her life and affection for her, she paused, and then said, "I guess he doesn't actually tell me he loves me. I really just assumed that."

Gradually it dawned on her that whenever she wanted his advice, he was willing to offer it, but she initiated the conversation. He did not pursue her. Further reflection made her aware of how uncertain she felt within their relationship. This uncertainty had been covered over by her telling herself that he loved her, despite her not hearing it directly from him. She eventually made the connection between how hard she worked to demonstrate her value and her deep longing for her father's approval—approval that she wanted to hear out loud with real words and physical gestures but seldom if ever did. Additionally, in her ascent from undergraduate to graduate school and then in the world of policy making, there had been a direct, fail-proof relationship between her hard work and being promoted. Her sense of adequacy was consistently tied to her effort, and when her effort did not change the course of her supervisor's behavior, her default conclusion was that something was wrong with her.

I mentioned that it was instructive that she had not spoken with her father about her situation, almost as if in so doing she would risk exposing her "failure" without the confidence that he would be comforting and reassuring. I asked what, ideally, she hoped he would do if she were to reveal her predicament to him. Tears formed immediately. "I love you, and you're going to be okay," she barely whispered.

This is not a story of gross abuse of power or abject neglect. Miriam's supervisor was indeed missing certain management skills and, as Miriam eventually discovered, felt no small amount of threat in her presence. But he was not a sociopath. Others' dramas are far worse. This is a First World problem, one could say. But it highlights two important features of being human. First, we can experience shame by virtue of what does *not* happen in our lives, in this case the lack of words and actions of affirmation on the part of Miriam's father. Second, like any of us, Miriam received the message, albeit subtly, that *she was at risk of being left if she did not work hard enough to prevent it*. At first glance, one might think this to be a ludicrous conclusion to draw. But we must recall that from a brain standpoint, at any given moment we are either moving generally toward or away from relationship with others or within ourselves. And to move away to any degree carries with it the potential risk of eventual abandonment. There is no more powerful siren call that warns us of this than shame. As such, any movement away without a clear indication of return—which is how Miriam's brain interpreted her father's silence—works harmonically with shame. Hence, not only does shame warn us of the potential of leaving, but leaving with no indication for the intention of reappearing also activates shame, even in deeply hidden and quiet ways outside our conscious awareness. Miriam's supervisor, while not necessarily intending it, not only shamed her in his interactive style but also activated within her the implicit memory of shame that had long been brewing between her and her father.

Thus, amid all the obvious story lines involved in Miriam's narrative—her boss's style, the need for her to have a conversation with him to define expectations and so on—shame percolated like a subterranean spring, feeding the emotional undercurrent of her story. Despite what appeared to others as obvious, logical solutions, Miriam's PFC was not regulating her life. Instead, her mind was constantly racing into an anticipated future in which she would be indefinitely imprisoned by the sensation and feeling of shame. She was not thinking this consciously and rationally, but rather sensing and imaging this as she drowned in the quicksand of emotion. This led not to straightforward interventions, such as a clarifying conversation with her boss, confident that she would land on her feet no matter what. Instead it led to anxiety, depression and a downward spiral of decreasing vocational creativity and engagement. Shame could not be more pleased with such an outcome.

## Starting to Make Sense of It All

For all of the off-putting features of shame we have explored thus far, we might wonder if there is ever a time when shame serves a helpful purpose.

Are we faithfully telling the whole story by only considering its negative attributes? For indeed the Bible suggests that shame can turn a person in a proper direction (e.g., Proverbs 19:26; 1 Corinthians 6:9).

As I mentioned earlier, there is a normal interpersonal neurobiological response that Schore has designated as the earliest evidence of shame. This response emerges from our developing autonomic nervous system enabling us, under a caregiver's attuned presence, to develop appropriate self-regulatory behavior. However, shame becomes a more complex problem when the attunement part of the equation—whether from parent, spouse, teacher, friend or employer—never arrives. Furthermore, as Dan Siegel points out, citing the work of Alan Sroufe, we frequently find ourselves in situations where shaming behavior is *intentionally* applied, even if nonconsciously.[13] It is to those situations of intentional application of shame—again, even if the behaviors are outside the conscious awareness of the one applying it—that the content of this book is directed.

In this chapter we have been exploring the multiple dimensions of shame as it operates within an interpersonal neurobiological framework. We were introduced to the primary task of developing joyful relationships that lead to the creative exploration and discovery of our world. We have observed shame's character as a powerful, unexpected emotional shift that catches us off-guard, leaving us with a deep sense of feeling cut off, pushed out and, in the worst moments, contemptible. In its wake is left the debris of broken dreams and lost relationships, the evidence of joy that has been unexpectedly sheared off. Harkening from chapter two, we can see that among other things, one of its signature features is its capacity to disintegrate systems, whether an individual mind, a relationship or whole communities and nations, isolating them from each other, with relational asphyxiation being the inevitable outcome. This can begin in our earliest relationships, but can extend into every relationship throughout the life cycle. It can occur in large, singular, traumatic events, or in repeated, everyday events that we barely notice and would not immediately associate with shame.

So far we have focused on the mechanics of shame—how it works. But what does that have to do with the soul of shame and the story it is trying to tell? Here we make the transition from *how* we operate as people who are fully embodied and fully relational to the *meaning* of what those interactions are about. From the perspective of IPNB we now turn to the narrative domain of integration, that realm of the mind in which, within the context of significant attachment relationships, we decide what is true about the world and our place in it. For as we will see in chapter four, storytelling is the feature that ultimately sets us apart from the rest of the earth's creatures—and the feature that shame intends to most powerfully exploit in order to lay waste to any attempts we would make to join God in creating a world of goodness and beauty.

# The Story of Shame
# You Are Living

It took him more than ten years to get to my office. Although he had considered seeing a psychiatrist on more than one occasion, it was not until his work was compromised that he felt compelled to take the plunge. Robert's depression had intensified over the previous six months to the point where acquaintances were worried about his welfare. He reported that he rarely left his apartment except to go to work, and he had little interest in being with his friends. "I have no motivation. I just want to feel better."

In our first meeting, in addition to the standard evaluation of his symptoms, we explored what life had been like growing up and who the important figures were that shaped what he understood to be the big picture of life. He acknowledged that he assumed his parents had been the primary influences on his life (although the specifics he couldn't name). But he was puzzled how this question had anything to do with why he had come to see me. He was depressed. What did that have to do with his notion of the meaning of life? Wasn't a lack of motivation a symptom of a mental disorder for which you could take some medicine and feel better?

This was a serious question on his part. He was clearly intelligent, to which his hefty paycheck as an actuary bore witness. But "the meaning of life" was something that he genuinely doubted had much to do with a brain disorder. Nothing he had read seemed to indicate Prozac and purpose had much to say to each other. I inquired about the nature, if any, of his spiritual practices. There were none, he reported. The words *spiritual practices* themselves sounded almost foreign to him. "My parents made me go to church when I was young, but I don't believe in any of that stuff anymore."

I wondered aloud about his reflections on where we came from and what is the purpose of life in general. I assured him that I was not attempting to find out about his belief in God. Rather, I was inquiring about what he believed about *anything*. Indeed, what was the story that—whether he attended to it consciously or not—was dominantly shaping the life he was embedded in?

He had trouble finding the words, more flummoxed than ever. "My story? I really have no idea."

Robert was aware that he was depressed. But he had no understanding that his disconnection from his own life story was feeding that depression. Symptoms were all he could see. He was blind to how the story he was telling with his life was bringing him to the brink of an emotional breakdown.

●●●

At the outset of this book I suggested that to know how shame works—its mechanics—can be helpful, but it is not enough to know this apart from knowing the story in which it occurs. For if we believe we live in a world created by the God whose character and acts are found in the pages of the Bible, then shame is no mere artifact. It has purpose in a larger narrative, an interpersonal neurobiological instrument that is intentionally and skillfully used to distract and disrupt the story God is telling. But how was shame playing a role in what Robert had shared with me thus far? Furthermore, how would understanding the nature of storytelling reveal not only the essence of shame's mechanics but also the way it influenced his story—and subsequently promoted the symptoms that brought him to my office?

We live our lives through the medium of stories. In order to become familiar with what shame is up to in the midst of the chronicles we are telling, it is instructive to be aware of some of the features of stories and storytelling. Shame wants to alter our stories by telling its own version, one that is sure to bring trouble wherever it goes.

## No Mere Tall Tale

As humans develop, we begin to do what to our knowledge no other animal does: we tell stories. We begin as newborns who are sensing, perceiving, imaging, feeling and moving, interacting with our inner and outer environments. We have to learn that our hands are our hands and that they can do things; we have to learn that our mother's voice belongs to our mother. We learn to walk and are drawn to eat the pansies. Eventually we acquire and develop the use of language. With words, we begin to use verbal (and then written) symbols to integrate our experiences, both in terms of how we interpret and communicate them to others. We become so proficient with language, in fact, that the nonverbal sensory data emerging from within and outside our mind-body matrices soon fades into the realm of nonconsciousness. These are not unavailable to us but are largely overtaken by the efficiency and effectiveness of language while simultaneously continuing to provide the fuel supply for the very words we are learning to use.

Therefore, we must be mindful from the outset that although we pay great attention to the language of stories as we tell them, a great deal of those stories unfold without words. Given that 60-90 percent of human communication is a function of nonverbal expression, it behooves us to pay attention to all that we say while leaving language out of the picture. Despite our sophistication in the use of language, which enables us to do the complex things we do, emotion and its regulation through sensations, feelings, imagery and physical movement still provides significant energy for our storytelling ventures. We don't necessarily have to have words to know that we are happy, sad or tormented. Words are extraordinarily helpful, but they are not the source of our torment. And so our narratives begin with sensations, images and feelings; merge into a word or thought; and end with *War and Peace* and *The Shawshank Redemption*.

This is critical in understanding how shame begins to weave its way into our lives. It does not wait for us to acquire language to insert itself. It primarily amounts to a shift in sensory-affective tone, an emotional shearing (see chap. 3). And with our first awareness of what we feel comes the potential for sensing shame, though we aren't old enough to have words to describe it as such. As Robert and I continued to talk over many weeks, he became more persuaded of the notion that his depression was not just a chemical imbalance. Indeed, though neurobiology was an important feature of his symptoms (one cannot separate matter from experience when it comes to the mind), as he reflected on his story, he began to connect the dots between his life growing up and his current state of affairs.

He recalled an early memory of his mother worrying about him (not least because of her own insecurities) whenever he had the opportunity to try new things, which made him feel uncomfortable and tentative. His father reacted to his mother's worry by at times overcompensating, forcing Robert to do things he was either not interested in or not ready for, which made him equally unsettled and caught in the crossfire of his parents. Notably, little direct, verbal commentary indicated that his parents thought he was inadequate. Neither parent came right out and said, "You don't have what it takes to survive in the world." Rather, Robert *felt* inadequate. There was never a time he could recall when he hadn't felt it. This is an example of how shame indirectly, in clandestine fashion, begins to weave its threads into our stories, accessing those parts of our brain that are, in the early years of our lives, most in charge: the brainstem, limbic circuitry and right hemisphere. Language, however, soon enough begins to support shame's efforts.

In the exploration of storytelling, if we were in the business of describing the mechanics of our development, we might say we are witnessing the progressive emergence of the complexity of interactions between different functions of the mind, which is true. But we are not merely becoming complex beings made up of random mental processes. Rather, within that complexity we are also making meaning. In other words, we eventually use words and everything else in our toolbox to make sense of—to tell the stories of—our lives. And in this way we not only acquire language, we also construct meaning. Our minds are at all times sifting and collating the various sensations, images, feelings, thoughts and behaviors we experience. With rhythmic periodicity our thoughts emerge, at times with intention and reflection, at others with impulsive automaticity, in order to make sense of or draw conclusions about those experiences, while in the process regulating emotion. This dance between these various elements of the mind is taking place ceaselessly and seamlessly throughout our day. We cannot *not* do this and live in this world. We can, however, be quite unaware that we *are* doing this.

Initially, Robert was aware of the winds blowing on the surface of his life, but not to the tectonic movements underneath. With time, he began to see how he used language to make sense of what he felt when shame became part of his embodied experience. He recalled how, when dealing with his mother's anxiety or his father's silence, thoughts and images would literally flash through his mind, and he would tell himself (though usually not out loud) things such as *I probably can't do that* or *I'll never make Dad happy.* In other words, he began to construct, even at an early age and without his knowing it, a narrative that as an adult would explain what he felt. For we use language, among other things, to help us solve problems by explaining and making sense of them. This making sense process includes not just the logical explanation of events but also an emotional shift toward a state of less distress. We don't want to know how things are because we are logical; our logic helps us regulate our emotion, which is the energy around which the brain organizes itself.

Hence, Robert not only "explains" things to himself through his narrative, he also regulates his emotional tone. One of the challenges this poses is that as I tell this version of my story repeatedly, I can draw the conclusion that my shame has its source in the very things I have been telling myself. For example, Robert's initial understanding for the reason he sensed shame was "because I'm really not that confident at things, especially relationships." In Robert's mind shame followed the "fact"—as he told himself—that he was inadequate. It had not occurred to him that his shame was not first a result of the story he told himself but rather its cause, its emotional source. It did not register with him that his parents' behavior was a source of what he experienced. Who wouldn't feel shame if the running undercurrent of your life included, if even in nearly undecipherable tones, the repeated *sense* that you are not enough?

We might conceptualize Robert's problem as one in which he believed a lie, an experience in which he absorbed a false reality. At one level, this is not untrue. But to believe anything, let alone a lie, is not a one-step mental process of engaging in a singular act we call "belief." For to believe something involves the mobilization of multiple realms of mental activity, including sensations, images, feelings, thoughts and physical behaviors, all of which converge mysteriously into what we eventually believe. For Robert, therefore, his conflict was not reducible to believing a lie; it was more complex than that. For he found himself quite unable to simply disbelieve the lie he had practiced believing for so long.

These chapters Robert wrote in his mind were not only his way of making sense of what he was feeling. They were also ways for him to cope, to reduce the noxious feeling of shame. How so? Recall that when it comes to emotional distress, especially something as off-putting as shame, the brain will do whatever it can to reduce that distress as expeditiously as possible. In this way our response to shame, whether turning away physically or constructing our narrative, only reinforces it. For in Robert's telling, he was also hearing that he was not enough. And with this we catch a glimpse of what evil is up to, using shame as its proxy. It wants us to tell our stories in such a way that *we* are the sole responsible party for what we feel; it wants us to live in isolation rather than in relationship. I feel shame, then, because I am shameful. I sense this because there is something wrong with me. It does not strike me that the reason I feel what I do is because of something that has happened *to* me as a function of my being in relationship with someone else. Despite my knowing as a fact that someone has said or done something to me that has evoked this awful feeling, shame's neurobiological tendency is that I quickly take personal ownership for it. But how could I possibly know this? I was so young when the whole process began.

## Macroscopic, Microscopic and Everything in Between

One rather simple way to think about our story is via the categories of large, medium and small. Our large story consists of what we think of in terms of metaphysics or a worldview. For instance (and not to oversimplify this), we either believe in God (or want to) or we don't, with all of its implications. We think our life has purpose or it doesn't. We think it's generally important to obey rules or we don't. Or perhaps some more ambiguously mixed version of any of these.

These are what I call macroscopic views of the world we live in, the world seen from ten thousand feet. It also includes various cultural memes and social ecologies that influence what we believe and how we act through multiple nonconscious (yet willful) interactions that we have with each other and with cultural artifacts such as art, technology or economics.

Our medium story, held within the large one, includes the details of our lives that are more particular to us within the context of the macroscopic world. In addition, it tends to represent lasting, salient emotional memory that we have implicitly encoded as part of our ongoing narration. These may include *I believe my father loves me. I don't believe my marriage will survive, let alone thrive. I'm worried I may lose my job. I'm so glad my son is finally dating someone. I love the New York Yankees. I hate the New York Yankees.* They represent threads of our mental life that, depending on the time of day, will hold varying degrees of sway and can shape moment-to-moment decisions that have lasting relational consequences.

Small or microscopic stories are ones that insert themselves in ways that are so temporary we barely notice them, and they may have little impact on our life. Or they could change our day completely. You are sitting in a conference and realize you should have used the bathroom before you came back for the late-afternoon session. Your mind drifts during a sermon as you wonder about the meal you have to prepare when you go home. You notice a hair out of place while looking in the mirror and move it back to where it belongs. You put your dirty cup in the dishwasher. You see a beautiful woman and fight to direct your image-making mind from where it wants to go.

I call these microscopic narratives not because they carry no gravitas but rather because of their general brevity. Notice too that what I have described in terms of storytelling is not to be constrained merely to thoughts we think or words we say. Our actions also tell our story. To put the cup away may include no conscious thought (although it could). The action, however, is no less your word.

These macroscopic, microscopic and in-between stories have no hierarchical status per se, and the borders between them are quite porous. The intended purpose of this model is simply to draw our awareness to the fact that we are engaged in the storytelling process at various levels simultaneously, each of them interacting with the others. And to the degree that we increase our awareness of these spheres, we equally become aware of when and how shame attempts to become part of our storytelling effort.

As Robert became progressively more open to and aware of these various spheres of his story, he discovered that shame was no respecter of any of them. He came to see how shame had the potential to taint virtually any moment of his storytelling process. When it joins us at early ages, and through the subtlety of nonverbal and verbal interactions, it becomes like a virus that spreads early and often until it infects the entire body. This does not mean that every single thought or image is a product of shame. However, it does reflect that shame does not limit itself to obvious parts of our story. It is not only the voice of our coach telling us we are the worst free-throw shooter she has ever seen. It is not restricted to the memory of the rape. No, it lives in our mind waiting for unexpected opportunities to color the feeling of a moment with its nondescript residue that we would barely identify as having anything to do with our subject.

## THE OPENING CREDITS

It may be revealing to know that telling your story begins with someone else. Long before you arrive on the scene, before and then after you were conceived, people started talking about you: they talked about your gender, what you will be named, who they hope you will resemble in appearance and character (and likewise, who they hope you will *not* resemble). And even before this, perhaps your parents had months or even years of longing for you. Or perhaps no one longed for you, and you were eventually passed on to someone else for your care. We are all born out of preludes of beauty and tragedy, each of us with our own ratio of both. You began your life out of and into this narrative that others were already telling.

But others' contribution to your narrative never stops. For even as we acquire language and mobility, growing in our independence and agency with the dawning awareness of our capacity to direct our own thoughts and respond to our own feelings, we are always interacting with other people. And their versions of the world—our world in particular—continue to shape and influence the way we understand and tell our unfolding narrative. First our parents, then teachers, friends, coaches, spouses, children, employers, employees and even panhandlers on the street are writing in the margins of our autobiographies. We are tempted to believe we are solo artists, but we are more like featured soloists in a symphony. The question, of course, is what kind of music we will play together.

As Robert came to see, his narrative actually had much older roots that began even before his parents were telling their own stories. His paternal grandfather had been a successful businessman who lost his life's earnings when swindled by someone he trusted. Thus Robert's father learned that trust is not entered into lightly. He worried about not being able to provide for his family, despite running his own successful accounting firm. Robert began to see that despite the appearance that his mother was the worrier in the family, his father merely translated worry into working harder to make sure he was self-sufficient, no matter how illusory that idea was. Their collective worry was shame telling them—and ultimately Robert—that in the end they will not be okay.

As this dawned on Robert, he made the connection to how hard he worked at work. Yes, because he enjoyed it (or had before he became depressed), but not without the undercurrent that he feared he would become the poster child for failure. He was able, with his logical brain, to see how this was not likely, but that fact was not swaying the emotional part of his brain, which was repeating the story he had received from his parents, a story about him others were telling before he was born.

## LISTENING TO TELL

Another way others participate in our storytelling is deeply rooted in the practice of listening. As we tell others our stories, to the degree they are helpfully attuned to us, our story is modified. The very act of attuning to someone nonverbally creates right hemisphere to right hemisphere brain connections that alter the experience in real time. In this way, good listeners energize the storyteller, and so encourage the story to be told more faithfully. They also ask good questions, and when necessary limit or redirect the speaker in order to get the best out of the story. Hence, storytelling is much more a dance between teller and listener than it is a monologue. In fact, it is fair to say that the story is what tends to emerge between speaker and listener, both playing a crucial role in its telling.

This is true even when we are having fleeting private thoughts. For no part of our story is not at some level being influenced by our experience with others, whether that person is in the room or not. Initially, Robert appeared uncomfortable with the level of attention I paid to him—his eye contact, his body movement, the less-than-audible voice. Eventually, when the time seemed proper, I offered reflections and observations on these things. Furthermore, as he told his story, pieces were obviously missing. If I did not inquire about the nature of his relationships, he would not speak of them. If I did not ask what he felt in his body when he described being anxious, he would not consider it important. Over time, however, he began to respond to queries about what he felt and how those feelings developed over the course of his life.

When we reached those instances of deep sadness and shame (as invariably is the case), his story began to change. It was transformed first by his awareness that these feelings were present and active. This was followed by his growing awareness that he had carried these feelings for much of his life but was only now engaging them with intention, but not by himself. The fact that he was telling his story to someone who (hopefully) was sharing that feeling with him changed how his brain was being wired and how his narrative was being rewritten. As he felt and reflected on his emotion in a shared relationship, its nature and his memory of it was changing. As such, his understanding—his story—of shame and of his life were being altered in the way of goodness and beauty.

Shame interferes with good listening at every level and every opportunity. How many times have I, while in conversation with someone, found myself only superficially attuned to what he or she is saying as I prepare what *I* want to say, sensing that if I do not get to offer my contribution I will feel a lessening? We all know this moment. We do not realize that shame is at work via the sensory networks by which I feel the urgency to speak rather than listen. In this way, shame is a shared process whose mission is to disrupt connection between people.

It was a novel idea to Robert that his emotional health had something to do with how well his parents and other significant attachment figures were listening, or not, to his story. Over time Robert began to explore the way his relationships, and in particular their attunement to him, had shaped not only his thoughts but also his sensations, images and feelings, along with his interpretation of them. He came to see that stories are never told in isolation but are always a collaborative affair, and that our dialogue partner may or may not be in the room with us. For even if my father has been deceased for several decades, I still hear his voice in my ear, smell his cologne and see him sitting in his favorite chair.

## QUALITIES OF GOOD STORIES

Good stories have beginnings, middles and ends. They emerge from somewhere and go somewhere. But unlike a book, whose words do not change over the course of years, our stories change routinely with the passage of time. When Peter was nineteen, his parents, David and Elena, informed him that his biological parents were the couple he had known all his life as his Uncle Max and Aunt Grace. The adults he had known as his parents, David and Elena, were in fact his aunt and uncle. When Peter entered the world, his biological parents had been too dysfunctional to raise him. His interactions with them over the course of his life consistently reflected this in their seeming lack of maturity in their decisions. When he had been born, all parties agreed that Max and Grace were not capable of raising Peter. Grace's sister, Elena, and her husband agreed to adopt him on the condition that confidences be kept until Peter was an adult. Needless to say, keeping the secret required great effort on all parties' parts. More to the point, the facts as Peter understood them changed overnight, as did his comprehension of his story.

Most of us don't have to endure the sort of whiplashing that Peter did, but the landscape of our stories do change in terms of the meaning we draw out of events we remember or anticipate. For instance, when we are teenagers our vision of what life was like as children may differ greatly from how we view that same time when we are in our fifties. Similarly, our anticipation of the future is powerfully influenced by the particular age we view it from.

For Peter, the changing of the "facts" was shame's opportunity to tell a different story beyond them. In Peter's mind, his capacity for predicting the nature of the world was turned on its head. How can I trust anyone? Moreover, how can I trust myself? If my closest family is willing to lie to me for so long over such important matters, who won't do the same? How can I know that anyone is who he or she claims to be? Peter underwent a comprehensive disorientation as these facts changed in his life. And in those moments of either minimal or catastrophic disorientation, we sense the feeling that something is deeply inadequate about us. Here we see how important it is for us to know our facts well, and not just as a means of doing things the right way (making sure I know that this medicine works but only in a certain dosing range), but as a way to fend off the potential for shame to mushroom into something much greater than I believe I can tolerate.

In Robert's case his initial rendition of his childhood began to shift as he learned more about how his mind worked, especially in response to parents who, doing the best they could, still had limitations that kept them from being present for Robert. It is common for people who are depressed to have a very different understanding of their past, as well as their future, compared to when they are well. Via neuroplasticity and Hebb's axiom, practice tends to make permanent. Thus, if we tell ourselves, using imagery and sensations as much as words, that our life isn't going anywhere, we literally wire our brain to continue in that pattern of storytelling. It becomes an embodied reality, and no amount of theological facts that state otherwise, apart from equally embodied action, will necessarily change the story's outcome. Robert began to see how the "facts" of his life were not immutable realities but were as much a function of the story he told himself on a moment-to-moment basis.

Another feature of stories is that we tell them in order for them to be heard. We don't find much meaning talking to the mirror or into thin air.

It is true that if we are wise we don't say everything that we think—there is great value in restraint. But when we are in the telling process, we long to be listened to. I don't like it when gathered with friends, for example, I am telling a story and in response to some distraction people stop paying attention, moving on instead to whatever has overtaken them in the moment. At first, this might seem obvious; no one likes to be ignored. But more to the point, it offers us a glimpse into at least some of the purpose of stories: they are a medium by which we are connected to others. In this sense I don't just tell a story, even a good one, for the sake of the story alone. Indeed, I tell it for my own sake, even if the story is not about me. I want to tell my story in no small part because I want to be known. For in so doing I experience what it means to be connected to people—which is what my brain longs for as much as anything.

## DEEP BENEATH THE SURFACE

In chapter two we reviewed the nine domains of integration as Daniel Siegel has described them. We noted that implicit memory enables us to move through our days without having to pay attention to every detail of activity. Otherwise it would be very difficult to walk and talk at the same time. Through this feature of implicit memory, we tell so much of our stories to ourselves and those around us—yet often without our conscious awareness. This represents the way that much of our story is nonconsciously narrated. When Robert became uncomfortable during our sessions, he would routinely and automatically fold his arms tightly across his chest. When I brought this to his attention he was unimpressed with its significance. But when I asked him to consider putting his arms at his side, he found this generated within him a greater awareness of his level of discomfort. "I guess I'm just nervous." Our dialogue eventually led to his recollection that this posture was one his father routinely maintained whenever he was speaking with Robert's mother and was not happy with the way the conversation was going.

Any time his father thought his mother was parenting Robert too softly, fearful that something would be too hard for him, Robert's father would sigh and cross his arms. Robert assumed this was his father's way of keeping from losing his temper, which had built over years in an uncommunicative marriage. Eventually Robert was able to tell me that he crossed his arms whenever he felt something—it could be anything—that was uncomfortable, but especially that needed to be contained. I wondered what message he thought he was sending to himself and to others with his action. "That I'm not safe, I guess." I asked him to conduct a simple experiment. He was to monitor the number of times in the course of one week that he crossed his arms when in a similar circumstance. It turned out that it happened several times a day. Without too much difficulty he realized that one of the main themes of the story he was telling was that he was not safe, that he was in relational and emotional danger. "Imagine what that would be like for you to have someone telling you that several times a day," I stated. The gravity of this nonconscious part of his story was not lost on him. The problem, of course, was learning how to tell a different one.

From Robert's life we see how so much of the story we are telling is coming from parts of us that are deeply buried, associated with neural networks from the brainstem, limbic circuitry, temporal lobes and right hemisphere, circuits whose activity are not associated with immediate conscious awareness. This does not mean, however, that we cannot become more aware of these shifts in neurobiological activity. Robert was only beginning to find out, and as he did, he also began to see the dominant role that shame played along the way.

Suffice to say, stories are told not just by individuals but by families, communities, churches and entire cultures. "We" believe certain things to be true, such as what is sacred and profane, what is to be protected and preserved, and what is to be judged, scorned or disposed of. This is a good thing when the story being told is one of redemption and wholeness. However, when shame is given the freedom to do its thing, isolation, condemnation and stasis are the result. It is one thing for me to experience the derision of my own internal voices, and yet another to hear the contempt of someone else. But when I perceive that I am receiving the shame from a community of voices, the pain can become unbearable. When the collection of the voices of an entire community shames us, it is much more unwieldy due to our inability to locate it centrally in any one place. And so when I feel shame in my family or my church, addressing it feels quite overwhelming.

## OUR SHAME ATTENDANT

Shame's presence is ubiquitous and inserts itself into the genetic material of the human storytelling endeavor. One way to envision shame is as a personal attendant. Imagine that you have a completely devoted attendant attuned to every sensation, image, feeling, thought and behavior you have. However, imagine that your shame attendant's intention is not good, is not to care for you but rather to infuse nonverbal and verbal elements of judgment into every moment of your life. The word *attendant* at first may seem counterintuitive, as it usually applies to someone who has our best interests in mind. But this is how shame works, a wolf disguised in sheep's clothing. Hence, our shame attendant appears in language, feelings, sensations and images that may on the surface seem acceptable, common and normal, but its purpose is anything but being helpful. We each have our own who attends to every turn in our storytelling venture, no matter how large or small the moment. Our attendant is waiting to offer advice, suggestions and reflections with the intended purpose of disintegration. Shame lurks in your bedroom, your wardrobe or your bathroom (especially the ones with really big mirrors). When we wake up each morning, our attendant greets us with the words "Wow, you really didn't get enough sleep last night. What were you thinking?" You move to the bathroom to take a shower and are reminded that you look like you have put on more weight.

You get in your car to go to work and your attendant whispers that the conversation you have scheduled with your difficult client is going to go poorly because you are ill-prepared. Later that day as you are bored at work and your mind drifts off to the beach where you would rather be, you hear that you won't ever have the job you really desire. While that is taking place, the shame attendants of each of your colleagues are also quite busy, deepening their reluctance to help others by reminding them that to do so will lessen their chance for advancement. In fact, as the attendant is quick to point out, no one in this company really cares about doing meaningful work. You may be the supervisor who is reminded by the attendant that you will not be okay if you do not make your quarterly quota. And of course, you won't be okay because your boss is listening to his attendant say the same thing.

When you arrive home, your wife, seemingly unworried about hiding any sense of resentment in her voice, reminds you of the leaking toilet, which you said you would repair two weekends ago. And the shame attendant, faithful as ever, offers you images of other failed handyman excursions, basting your mind in the notion that you are a mechanical moron. This does not give you more confidence, leading to feeling deflated and passive. All of which means, of course, that you are not likely to have sex with your wife tonight because she's not very attracted to a deflated, passive husband. And the attendant watches you, offering multiple opportunities to assimilate a story that tells you, in essence, that you are not enough, you do not have what it takes to be okay.

Or the attendant whispers that in the face of the emotionally and sexually abusive relationships you have had, no man would want you. Who would when they find out that you are damaged goods? Then there is the middle school geography teacher who worries that her students will not demonstrate enough progress this year, and so she becomes the voice of the attendant in the ears of her students, reminding them of their poor performance. Not because she wants to be a conduit of shame but because she is attempting to cope with her own sense of inadequacy.

As we have learned, part of the problem with shame and storytelling is that a great deal of my story is being told nonconsciously, albeit willfully. The teacher does not wake up in the morning *intending* to listen to the shame attendant. And for many of us, we may not be aware of any moments when the attendant is noticeable. And this is the point. Most of shame's activity in our stories does not take place in grossly evident events but rather in the accumulation of small moments: you step out of the shower into the light and reflection of the mirror, or think about the conversation you had with your spouse earlier and sense his disinterest in your feelings. In these ultrathin slices of time we co-construct, in partnership with our attendant, the story that shame wants to tell. And its nature is that it will not necessarily present itself in the front and center of your story, but rather off to the side, distracting you just enough to be nettlesome but not to draw your attention to it so much that you might actually do something about it.

Maggie had just about anything a woman could want. Married for more than three decades to a husband who was devoted to her, the mother of three children and the grandmother of two. And she had the distinct honor of being hired as the CEO of one of the top software engineering companies in the region. The board of directors had hired her explicitly to change the culture of the firm and to position them well for a desired initial public offering. This she had done well. But along the way she felt disrespected by a group of employees who worked in one division of the company. They were the only team who seemed to respond slowly to her leadership and balked at some of the innovations she wanted to implement.

But instead of addressing this group directly, she avoided conflict with them. Given all of her obvious leadership skills, how was this possible, and what role did shame play in her story? As we say in the business, we always take our family of origin with us to work, and Maggie took hers. She grew up in a setting where, despite her intelligence, there had never been much attention paid to her academic accomplishments, and life in her home was much more dedicated to the care of her special needs sibling, two years her junior. So much of her life had been consumed by meeting the needs of her younger brother that her interests had largely been ignored. Whenever she tried to express legitimate desires, she was met with unmitigated impatience or irritability. She learned to wire together in her mind the desire for being seen with the inevitable outcome of harsh belligerence.

Over the years, not surprisingly, in order to meet her needs Maggie learned how to work hard to make people happy. This, along with her intelligence, had won her many friends and led to the life she knew. But whenever she was confronted with someone who was uncooperative, she became fearful, tentative and accommodating. Little did she know that the shame attendant who had been active while she was growing up was now telling her that she could not tolerate what might happen if she confronted the uncooperative group in her workplace. Virtually everyone in her company overwhelmingly affirmed her work; shame did not present itself directly to her. Instead, it came in the side door through a small but vocal and passively resistant group of people who needed boundaries and direction—or termination. Although Maggie was able in the abstract to see that their behavior was not acceptable, her only way of seeing how to solve the problem was to work harder to change *her* behavior rather than to expect them to change theirs. She told herself that if she worked harder she would convince them to change. Shame may not come to us directly, but it always makes us feel solely responsible for the problem.

In this chapter we have explored some of the features of storytelling and have seen that telling stories is an inevitable characteristic of what it means to be human. We have also seen some of the ways that shame shapes our narratives. It is one thing to describe the nature of storytelling. It is quite another, however, to come to terms with which story we are actually living in. It is good to examine from a distance the nature of how stories are told and the different ways shame might influence that process. But to actually live in those stories is quite another matter. Some people, for instance, believed the world was flat. Most of us now believe the world is round. Which story you believe may not make much difference if you are a farmer in Iowa or Kazakhstan, but it matters a great deal if you are an engineer launching people into space. This is no different when it comes to shame.

If we want to be part of God's work in creating goodness and beauty in a world that is experiencing entropy, it is important to know which story you are actually living in. We may think we know, but our lives often betray that belief. In this light, we now will explore the biblical story of shame, and eventually catch a glimpse of the action God is taking to transform it.

# Shame and the
# Biblical Narrative

We have just explored the nature of storytelling and its importance in the way we encounter shame. We have discovered that to understand shame is not a purely academic exercise targeting an abstract topic. Shame is not only something that we weave in and out of our stories, describing it as we experience it, but something that actively, intentionally attempts to shape the stories we are telling. It is dynamic and fluid, changing its shape and consistency to fit the situation in which it finds us in order to dismantle every effort toward goodness and beauty that we desire to co-construct with God.

To combat shame we act in such a way that we live more robust, more confident and more creative stories. Such stories take greater risks of mercy and justice, which naturally make us more vulnerable. For the most human acts of creativity include the willingness to put the products of creation on public display, where they can be embraced or rejected. This includes everything from making babies to making bread, from painting houses to painting pictures, from leading people on a software engineering project to leading the choir in a rendition of Handel's *Messiah*.

Which story do you believe you are living in? As we discovered in chapter four, this may be one of the most important questions we ever ask ourselves. This chapter explores how the Bible's story views shame and its place in that narrative. Although we do not have the space here to discuss the anthropology that informs this exploration, it is important to be aware that the Bible tells a very different story about the nature of

our origins than does our present culture. Therefore, as Peter Berger and
Lesslie Newbigin attest, we must be careful and wise regarding the tacit
cultural assumptions that shape the stories of our lives that we tell.[1]

From the first pages of Genesis we read of a God of intention, a God
who has begun a story with a particular intended outcome. It is a story
that has direction and meaning given to it by the storyteller. But in this
same story there are other voices, and we are interested in one voice in
particular. A voice of evil, who has a very different intention than God
does. Its intention is to twist and sully the story of joy and creativity that
God is working so hard to tell. And I suggest that evil's maleficent intent
is wielded no more forcefully (yet subtly as part of its tactical prowess)
than through the use of shame. Within a biblical anthropology, shame is
not a neutral player on the field. It is not a mere artifact of our existence
or simply one of many different emotional states that emerge from our
neural networks.

## A BIBLICAL OFFERING OF SHAME

Elsewhere I have explored the emergence of shame in the history of humankind's origins as reflected in the biblical narrative.[2] Here we will
review the connections between shame, interpersonal neurobiology and
the way we tell stories about ourselves, each other and God. We will
touch on what I consider to be helpful parts of the story that contribute
to our goal of understanding shame and putting it to death. My intent is
to awaken your curiosity about what God was up to in the beginning and
how that is relevant for what we do in response to shame when we engage
a friend, employee, spouse or child. If we do not understand our history
of how shame has come to be our partner in life, we are, as George San-
tayana reflected, condemned to repeat it.

At the conclusion of Genesis 2, we have reached the culmination of
creation. All of material creation has been assigned its function (Genesis 1)
and name (Genesis 2). It has been duly noted that the God of this story
intends that the world will be one of joyful discovery, and for the cap-
stone—humankind—to live in communion with God and each other in
order to exercise creative dominion over it. So what's the point of the last

verse of chapter 2: "Adam and his wife were both naked, and they felt no shame" (v. 25)?

The writer has my attention. He could have chosen from an entire panoply of words or phrases to describe humankind's emotional state at this point. He could have said the man and woman were naked and really happy (who wouldn't be?), or they were naked and strong or confident, or they were naked and without fear or anger or sadness or disappointment or regret. And to be certain, all of these may have been true. With so many to choose from, why the emphasis on shame? It would seem that it is no accident.

We could argue that the writer inserts it as an afterthought to what transpires only a few lines later, giving the reader an anchor for what unfolds in Genesis 3. This may be the case, but I would suggest that shame's mention—juxtaposed to humankind's nakedness—is significant not simply because of what follows but also, and perhaps mostly, because it is *primal* to what follows. The vulnerability of nakedness is the antithesis of shame. We are maximally creative when we are simultaneously maximally vulnerable and intimately connected, and evil knows this. To twist goodness into the seven deadliest versions of its opposite, shame is necessary and effective, and its virulence explicitly exploits our vulnerability.

In other words, Genesis 2:25 is not just a passing description of humankind before Genesis 3. It is drawing our attention to the emotional fulcrum around which the history of sin rotates, the fundamental source, harbinger and herald of what is to come. I would suggest that the writer wants us to pay attention to shame not just because it happens to show up later but because of its central role in all that ends in a curse. It is *the* emotional feature out of which all that we call sin emerges. As such, in the biblical narrative when we experience shame, we are not simply encountering one of an array of possible emotions; rather we are engaging evil in its most fundamental mode of operation. This is not unlike C. S. Lewis's sense of the place of this emotion in our day-to-day lives: "I sometimes think that shame, mere awkward, senseless shame, does as much towards preventing good acts and straightforward happiness as any of our vices can do."[3] To the degree that we are aware of this and take

steps to properly respond to it, we more effectively become more connected, courageous and creative in whatever domain we occupy.

## DESCENT INTO HELL

In *Anatomy of the Soul* I suggest a way to consider how the encounter in
Genesis 3 might unfold. Here I will briefly recapitulate those reflections.
But first a word of caution. We must always be careful not to project our
own psychological interpretations, where it is not warranted, into any
story in which we are not direct participants, not least that of Scripture.
That is even more true when little if any explicit mention is made of what
is coursing though the minds of the characters involved. However, really
good stories—and this is a good one—tend to compel our curiosity
about what the characters are thinking, feeling, sensing and so on. To
refrain completely from considering the workings of the inner lives of
Eve and Adam ultimately leaves us unable to relate to them in any meaningful ways, for surely what we do is an extension of our inner life, as
Jesus himself reminds us (Matthew 15). I offer these reflections as an
invitation to consider how shame is wielded as the primary tool by which
evil has been doing its business from the very beginning—and as an
invitation to know who we are *now*, not just who we were *then*.

The text opens with a dialogue between a serpent and the woman.

> Now the serpent was more crafty than any of the wild animals the
> LORD God had made. He said to the woman, "Did God really say,
> 'You must not eat from any tree in the garden'?"
>
> The woman said to the serpent, "We may eat fruit from the trees
> in the garden, but God did say, 'You must not eat fruit from the tree
> that is in the middle of the garden, and you must not touch it, or
> you will die.'"
>
> "You will not certainly die," the serpent said to the woman. "For
> God knows that when you eat from it your eyes will be opened, and
> you will be like God, knowing good and evil." (Genesis 3:1-5)

We note, among other things, that the creature we are introduced to
is *crafty*. Other translators offer the word *subtle* instead of *crafty*. Each

has distinct value in describing the creature's nature. The general sense is that he, this *nachash* (Hebrew for "burning one" or "bright one"), was the wisest of all the creatures God had made. But the implication, given the context of the story, is that his wisdom is "crafty" in the sense of being darkly shrewd. Its intention is to fool the woman. And to be fooled is to be shamed, if even at the subtlest nonconscious level of awareness. But we know this only because we know the end of the story. I would not necessarily have comprehended this any earlier than the woman did had I been in her shoes.

The creature and the woman engage in a conversation that activates several emotional shifts within the woman. His initial query introduces the possibility for doubt to enter the woman's mental framework. Doubt not only about God ("Did God really say . . . ?") but also about her recollection of history and by extension—and more importantly—doubt about the nature of her *relationship* with God. As Michael Polanyi has pointed out, in order for us to doubt anything, at the moment we do we simultaneously put our trust in something else.[4] We are invariably made for faith, to operate out of a need to trust something we cannot control.

Here we begin to see how shame works. By implication of the story's context, the serpent's question necessarily invites Eve to sort out the answer *by herself*. There is no indication that the creature was truly interested in acquiring information. Nowhere does the serpent suggest they go to God to check the facts. He is not at all concerned with the truth as a set of facts. He is far more interested in disrupting the relationships between the woman, God and the man. And speaking of the man, it would appear that, given his presence (v. 6) (whether during her conversation with the serpent or after), he does little to help the situation by remaining (stereotypically) silent on the matter of her encounter with the serpent.

Doubt is one of the more common occurrences in the human experience, one that has various levels of emotional intensity, depending on the topic at hand. Doubting that my favorite team will win the playoffs feels dissimilar to doubting that my child will survive a serious medical illness. However, each involves the reality that I am inadequate on my own—I am not enough—to guarantee the outcome I desire. This dynamic is constantly in play within and between us. We doubt the security of our job; that our marriage will survive, let alone thrive; that my child will be able to handle life in this complex world; that we are smart enough, attractive enough, funny enough. Or we may doubt that there is a God, let alone one who is with and for us. Doubt, though concerned with facts, is not primarily about them but rather about our emotional sensation of connection, security and confidence. It is noteworthy that we often attempt to solve our problems of doubt by acquiring more information—and this is not to be despised. If we doubt our knowledge of the proper medication to give to a patient, it is a good thing to double check. In this sense, doubt is a mental function that serves the purpose of our greater good.

But there is a darker side to doubt, and the serpent in Genesis 3 has every intention of exploiting it. In this scene, doubt is planted as a way to discredit not so much Eve's rendition of the facts, which could easily be resolved by waiting for God's next stroll through the garden. It is used to rupture relational connections. It is one thing to use doubt in the service of creating goodness and beauty, and of enriching relationships. It is quite another to do the opposite. So often when we doubt ourselves, especially in the face of what we consider to be important events in our lives, we are actually doubting our sense of connection with others, not least with God. We doubt that we will be okay. To be okay as a human is first and foremost about being connected to God and others. It is not ultimately about having enough information, skill, intelligence or experience. Neither is it about being youthful, svelte or ripped, nor having enough money, sex or power. And when doubt involves any of these, you can be confident that shame is the emotional feature that is deeply at work.

In Eve's response to the serpent, our attention is drawn to how things are changing. This shift in Eve's sensations, images, feelings and thoughts are a combination of the activation of her analytic, left-brain activity fueled by the emotional distress emanating from her limbic/amygdala and brainstem regions of her brain. Initially, this does not have to be overwhelming, but it does not require much to change ever so slightly the direction she is headed. Her answer to the serpent's question is revealing.

In verses 2-3 we see that the woman's version of history has been distorted. As far as we are aware, she offers a different rendition than the one God offered to Adam, the presumed source of what Eve would know about the tree and its fruit. Again, with Adam present, there would be ample opportunity for him to be helpful in the conversation. There is no evidence in the text that this happens. The discomfort that accompanies the early onset of doubt can foster this alteration of memory, and it happens all the time in our daily interactions. How many times have I changed my remembered version of an interaction with someone when my underlying sense of confidence has been shaken if only ever so slightly? This is a hallmark feature of shame's activity. It reflects the distress of a disintegrating process that is not unlike what we explored in chapter two. In the same way that an infant's trajectory of joy is interrupted or sheared off, even in slight ways, so also the interchange between the woman and the serpent portends the coming disintegrating storm. And we see this in every arena of interaction with ourselves and others.

Whether it was Adam or Eve who lost the facts in translation, it remains that this emotional wrinkle sets the stage for the serpent's next move. In the subtlest yet most provocative initiative yet, he twists the knife, activating more directly the dynamic of shame. As you read verses 4-5 of Genesis 3, consider for a moment what you *feel*. Refrain from the urge to read merely the facts offered to Eve; rather, imagine how the creature would likely appear and sound, and then look closely at the implicit message he is delivering.

In stating flatly that the woman will not die, the serpent offers her a new rendition of the truth. A startling one, to be sure. But this is not merely a factual sleight of hand. To be told that you will be like God may seem like a good thing. I would love to hear that. But the subtle corollary to this idea is that, given the prohibition to the fruit of this particular tree, by implication *God does not want you to be like him*. God does not want you to have what he has. He does not want you to be as close and as connected to him as you might think he does. And by further implication, therefore, *you are not as important as you think*. You, as it turns out, are *less than you think*. You. Are. Not. Enough.

This is not stated directly. To do so would be insufficiently subtle, too easily dismissed by the woman as she marshals her factual defenses.

Better to let the distressing affect of her doubt do the work. Recall that shame is primarily an emotion that undermines us not so much via our left-mode, rational processing but by eroding our *felt sense* of connection and safety, something that supersedes the linguistic, logical, linear, factual mode of mental activity. As such, in brain time, to be less than, to be inadequate, is felt, sensed and imaged long before we think it.

We also see that the serpent has no trouble talking *about* God rather than inviting the woman to have a conversation *with* God. This is one of shame's most important means of creating the isolation that supports its affective gravitas. At this point the woman can begin to consider God in her own mind, by herself. She is given the opportunity to decide independently who God is and what he thinks and feels in response to her. She begins the process of analyzing God—of judging him from a distance, rather than interacting with him. How many times do I do this in the course of a day? It is so easy to analyze, to judge, in the privacy of my own mind, what my friend, my enemy, my spouse, my child, my employee, my boss, my pastor, the person who just cut me off in traffic, the school board member, or the person of the other culture or religious tradition is really thinking or feeling. Often this judgment is not made first as a function of logical, language-based cognition. Rather, it emerges from the brain stem and limbic circuitry as something I sense and feel subtly but effectively. In so doing, it bypasses my logical, thinking brain such that I am hardly aware that judgment is even taking place. Before I know it, shame has taken root while I am oblivious to its presence.

Of course, the most effective—and possibly the supremely threatening—way to prevent the slide into this trap is to talk *with* God, rather than *about* him. But this idea never gains an audience in the Genesis story. And as we know, to relationally confront our shame requires that we risk feeling it on the way to its healing. This is no easy task. This is the common undercurrent of virtually all of our relational brokenness. We sense, image, feel and think all sorts of things that we never say, because we're far too frightened to be that honest, that vulnerable. But honest vulnerability is the key to both healing shame—and its inevitably anticipated hellish outcome of abandonment—and preventing it from taking further root in our relationships and culture.

The serpent adds that Eve's eyes will be opened by eating of the fruit of the tree of the knowledge of good and evil. Notice that he does not say that she will open her eyes, an act of intention on her part, but rather that they will be opened by someone or something else. What irony, in seeking to become like God she seems to miss the point that it will require something outside of her to provide what she is looking for. In my quest to become master of the universe, I too fail to see that to acquire what I am searching for always requires the assistance of something outside of me.

One way to read this is to assume that the creature hoodwinks the woman, enticing her to take hold of what she does not have. But it strikes me as odd that she would want what the serpent is offering unless she has already developed an underlying emotional distress she needs an antidote for. If the relationships between the man, the woman and God are unsullied, what else would she possibly desire? God has already given the couple the entire fruit of the garden to choose from—so much goodness—what else could they possibly want? I assume that before her encounter with the serpent, the woman has lived in a world of anticipated joy. She assumed she was loved and did not need to wonder about it, in the same way she did not need to think about breathing. That is, unless or until something comes along to interrupt it, to shear it off.

Here is where the primal emotional evocation of shame, from which proceeds all that we call sin, emerges. And all sin, all idolatry, all coping strategies in which I indulge are ways for me to satiate my hunger for relationship, my longing to be known and loved, my desire to be desired. Here, via the subtlety that only the craftiest wisdom can muster, the woman is accused of being undesirable, not enough. And as a solution for this the creature turns Eve's attention to the most desirable thing in the garden, which has nothing to do with relationship. Between the creature's initial question and his statement that reframes the woman's imagined reality, it is not too much to assume that shame is already working its magic long before she eats the fruit.

Here it is worth mentioning that the biblical narrative does not leave room for the woman's emotional state to emerge as a random artifact of evolution's developmental processes. It does not care about that. In Genesis, shame does not just happen apart from her interaction with a provocateur. In *this* story, which begins in a garden and is consummated in Jesus, it doesn't matter so much how the neuropsychiatric phenomenon of shame developed over how many hundreds of thousands of years. What matters is how it is used and how we respond to it when we experience it. Shame is not a mere sensation to be categorized in the same way that we would, say, an itch on my elbow. Here it is being wielded *with intention* for the purpose of ruining the world. It requires the activity of the serpent to start this process. In other words, the woman's underlying emotional distress does not happen without help from Mr. Crafty. It is a hallmark of shame that though I experience it as something being fundamentally wrong with me, I draw that conclusion only as a byproduct of my emotional sense of it as a harbinger of abandonment, as a function of the potential for a catastrophic rupture in relationship.

It is from this posture of emotional dysregulation and relational disintegration, under the guidance of shame, that Genesis 3:6 naturally follows.

> When the woman saw that the fruit of the tree was good for food and pleasing to the eye, and also desirable for gaining wisdom, she took some and ate it. She also gave some to her husband, who was with her, and he ate it.

In order for her to cope with her distress, the woman begins the analytic, left-brain-dominant mode of retelling the story of the tree at the center of the garden. Now, in the new narrative, instead of it being off-limits and the source of death by alienation, it becomes the potential source of life. Now she is able to tell her story without involving anyone else. No one else to make a mess of her life. No more disappointment. No more regret. No more hurt. No more limits. No more coauthors to contend with. It is far easier to live with a tree that is planted and fixed than with a God who can come and go as he pleases, leaving her vulnerable to a snake.

More explicitly, the fruit of this tree becomes the source by which she can cope with the mounting wave of emotional distress, her awareness of her inadequacy, her isolation, her shame. And the new narrative she constructs (with all the imagined benefits while disregarding the cost) becomes the way she retells her story—and foretells yours and mine—all the while reinforcing, rather than resolving, the emotional and relational disintegration that was the source of her appetite in the first place.

Shame has led to her replacing relationship with a pear. She walks away from engagement with Adam or God—a neurobiological state of "we"—and into the dark, blind alley of independence, all as a way of regulating the emotional disruption that has been introduced by her interchange with the serpent. Furthermore, it is no small thing that Adam apparently did nothing to intervene. We could speculate any number of reasons for this, but suffice to say, this fruit feast was a group effort, for at the very least Adam loaned his tacit approval.

It is so like shame to do this. By activating neural networks in our lower brain domains, it seeks to unconsciously and powerfully draw into its destructive vortex other individuals who are intimately associated with one in its grip. We witness the demeaning of a colleague by a supervisor and feel paralyzed to speak up. We know our spouse drinks too much but find ourselves unwittingly enabling his or her behavior. We seamlessly join a conversation criticizing a family member, coworker or parishioner as a way to mitigate our own distress that has been creeping just below the surface of our consciousness, waiting for the opportunity for release. We are deceived by the false sense of connection that temporarily holds sway over the small group gathered around the water cooler, or after church, to pass judgment on the target du jour. The work of shame can become so socially embedded after years and generations of practice that we are completely unaware of how we passively support the mistreatment of the other.

## DOWNLOADING THE VIRUS

The propagation of shame, when not relationally resolved, inevitably is made complete: "Then the eyes of both of them were opened, and they realized they were naked; so they sewed fig leaves together and made coverings for themselves" (Genesis 3:7).

The highlight of this text is the fact that the eyes of the man and woman *were opened*. Who or what is opening their eyes if they are not actively doing so? Could it be that each now sees the other in ways that are judging, condescending and extensions of what the woman took in from the serpent? In the same way that the woman's eyes are opened by the serpent, so this vector is transmitted to each other. In so doing, they became acutely aware of their nakedness, their vulnerability. Imagine the conversation: "So, Eve, I've noticed you have put on a few pounds." She retorts, glancing below his waist, "Perhaps, but I'm not nearly as unattractive as, well, *that*." Fig leaves are all they have left to cope.

After they have cut parts of each other out of their lives, they next do the same with God. "Then the man and his wife heard the sound of the LORD God as he was walking in the garden in the cool of the day, and they hid from the LORD God among the trees of the garden" (Genesis 3:8).

Hiding is the natural response to shame. This is especially true when we experience it in a toxic form, but most of our hiding takes place in the everyday comings and goings of life. We hide from everyone, not least being ourselves, in every imaginable way. Furthermore, all the hiding I do from others begins with all the smoke and mirrors I employ within my own mind. There are multiple parts of myself that I don't *want* to know. It would be too shaming. For I know the parts of me that I don't like, and that I presume that God does not either. They include my judging, lying, stealing, gluttonous, hoarding, lusting, adulterous, arrogant selves just to name a few. But as David Benner points out, quoting John Calvin, we cannot expect to know God fully if we are not willing to know ourselves, for one depends on the other.[5]

Hiding from my different parts, however, is just the beginning. All other secrecy is merely an extension of that. We hide from family members. We hide from those sitting next to us in the church pew. We hide from our spouse. We hide from our neighbors. We hide from other ethnic and religious groups. We live in a culture where we are afraid to reveal who we are for fear of being shamed for being who we are. We find it virtually impossible to have public discourse about anything that touches our more vulnerable parts. This hiding comes not only because we anticipate that we *will* be shamed, but even more important, in our memory we carry a sense that we *are* shameful. We walk on the earth burdened with the ancient code that we received from our first parents. We hide behind our rhetoric, and have come to depend on our various garments to protect us not so much from the *other* but from ourselves. When I am in the presence of another who elicits discomfort within me, though I easily point to the person outside my skin as the responsible party for my distress, the real problem is far more proximate. For it is ultimately within me.

My "problem," as it turns out, is ultimately what *I* am sensing, imaging, feeling, thinking and doing. It is not my only problem, just my ultimate one. This is not to say that someone else may not be *a* problem for me, or that if someone robs me or hurts my child my distress is only a function of my own mind. Rather it identifies where the ultimate source of my distress lies: within my own mind.

But beyond this, and even more important, my problem is not just what I am sensing but that I do not feel adequate to respond to it. I perceive, beginning at nonconscious levels of awareness, that I do not have what it takes to tolerate what I feel. I am not just sad, angry or lonely. But ultimately these feelings rest on the bedrock that I am alone with what I feel, and no one is coming to my aid. Shame undergirds other affective states because of its relationship to being left. And to be abandoned ultimately is to be in hell. This terror of being alone drives my shame-based behavior and, ironically, takes me to the very place I most fear going—to the hell of absolute isolation.

The first couple, disconnected and hiding from one another, have little if any reserve left to call on God when he comes walking into the cool of their day. Notice how shame gathers inertia as the couple hides together from God. This is one of shame's most powerful characteristics. When it lassos a group of people, shifting from its individual to corporate expression, shame's energy and intensity expands geometrically, the whole of its presence becoming far greater than the sum of its individual parts. The group's capacity for vulnerability shrinks, and the notion of being known disappears in favor of the need for protection from the very members that compose it. The community of faith that began in Genesis 2 now devolves, running into the woods.

God's relationship with the man and woman has not been as a casual bystander, but rather his presence is necessary for them to experience the joy they have presumably known. To live "in our image" would include God being present as a third party in the same way God lives in a triune fashion within himself. To cut God out of the equation necessarily enacts an inevitable countdown to relational implosion. But God does not give up on them, and instead comes calling.

> But the LORD God called to the man, "Where are you?"
>
> He answered, "I heard you in the garden, and I was afraid because I was naked; so I hid."
>
> And he said, "Who told you that you were naked? Have you eaten from the tree that I commanded you not to eat from?"
>
> The man said, "The woman you put here with me—she gave me some fruit from the tree, and I ate it."
>
> Then the LORD God said to the woman, "What is this you have done?"
>
> The woman said, "The serpent deceived me, and I ate." (Genesis 3:9-13)

The writer of the story does not presume that God is geographically challenged. God is inquiring of the couple's internal, not their external, whereabouts. He is deeply curious about and invested in their individual and corporate state(s) of mind. This is what the God of the biblical narrative does. He pursues. He comes to find us. Our perception is often of his walking away, leaving us out of his mind. Perhaps that tells us more about our perceptual capacity than his movement and presence. For in this story, his movement creates space for the woman and man to encounter their own and each other's inner selves in fresh, albeit challenging, ways, giving them the opportunity to confront what loving is all about—choosing *for* rather than *against* relationship in the face of shame's distressing presence.

God's inquiry appears genuine. There is no immediate evidence that it is offered in an accusing manner: "I know what you've done, and now you have hell to pay!" Given the context of the whole story, especially the intimacy with which God approached his creation in Genesis 2, it is reasonable to assume that there may be urgency in his step and his voice, given his longing for connection with the couple and his awareness that it is already teetering on the brink of extinction, but accusation is not to be found.

God's call is met with the man's admission that (1) he hid because (2) he was afraid because (3) he was naked (v. 10). The progression from 1 to 3 is the simple, universal cycle of shame we all experience. We inhabit a world in which we have inherited, genetically, epigenetically, generationally and culturally, the tendency to hide in response to the fear that is evoked by awakening to our vulnerability. But not simply our vulnerability as a *fact* but rather the *felt* implication of shame that heralds the impending abandonment we are about to undergo. Notice that fear follows the anticipation of the feeling of shame: "I was afraid because I was naked." Adam's felt sense of vulnerability—expressed as shame—drives the engine of the story as it unfolds. And so it is with all of us. Our vulnerability, ultimately to potential abandonment (of which shame is the herald), is simultaneously both the source of all that is broken in our world as well as its redemption.

## The Answer to the Question: Relationship

A curious thing happens next in verse 11. God's next comment is again a question, but not one I would necessarily expect. He does not ask *what*. He asks *who*. If I suspect that someone has done something they were prohibited from doing, I would certainly be more interested in the *what*. If I were God, I don't think I would have led with the *who* question. I mean, isn't the most important thing here whether the man has kept the rule? Isn't it important to teach them right from wrong? Isn't it important for them to answer for their mistakes? Perhaps.

Despite the fact that God quickly follows his *who* question with a *what* question, he approaches the problem as one that has its source primarily in the emotional context of relationship. He asks who informed the man and woman that they were naked. Is this not a nod to how our shame is relationally leveraged? An invitation to solve the matter together, rela-tionally, rather than by themselves? The next query, albeit about behavior, invites the man into dialogue. "Have you eaten from the tree?" A simple yes or no would do. But the horse of shame has left the barn, and the man and woman respectively do what we all have a tendency to do when we are genuinely sought, even when sought in love. Our shame screams out in judgment of those closest to us. Sure, it is easy and common for us to judge those who are the furthest from us. But we reserve our most ven-omous moments for those that circle most closely in our relational orbits. The man condemns the woman, and the woman follows suit, leaving God with the task of telling it like it is and like it will be for people and the creation alike. Sure, there is that prediction about the ultimate destiny of the serpent at the heel of God's Man in some unknown distant future. But for the moment, indeed for all our moments, it looks like evil has won.

Gone is the joy, which has been sheared off while the man and woman were not paying attention to what they were sensing, imaging, feeling or thinking. Disintegrated are the relationships in which God and the couple enjoyed the love of being known. It matters not that God attempts to engage the man and the woman, looking for a real conversation, a real partner in a real relationship. Shame would have none of that. No longer would connection, curiosity and creativity be engaged freely, without the worry of failure or of being exposed and humiliated for making mistakes. There was a new, bent order, one filled with thistles, undermining and abuse. Shame's mission was complete.

## FROM GOD'S STORY TO OUR STORY

So, to review: the opening of the story of the Bible reveals a God who creates with joy and intention, and who longs to have relationship with and be known by humankind. We see that he desires people to live as he lives, further exploring, stewarding and creating within the world. This is re-flected in what we know about the interpersonal neurobiological devel-opment of the mind, the place of joy as a principal feature in the growth of relationship, and the rhythm between connection (a secure base of re-lationship) and creativity (curiosity and exploration). These realities represent the teleological framework of the Bible's story. They characterize the foremost longings of our hearts in every domain of life we occupy.

The fingerprints of God's intention cover every square inch of our experience. We thirst for deep connection in our families, churches and yes in our workplaces. We deeply desire, even if we are not conscious of it, to be able to explore new things without worrying about making mistakes. We want to walk into a room without the anxiety of not being attractive, interesting or funny enough. We want to go to school and learn because we yearn for discovery, not because we worry we won't get into the best college, yet another blot on my record that reminds me I am not enough. We want to parent our children in ways that provide opportunity for growth without the understated, let alone blatant, message that they are not meeting our expectations. We want to tackle meaningful, hard conversations in our communities of faith about human origins or sexuality or economics without bracing against the specter of accusation. We long for our politicians to govern with curiosity, justice and mercy, rather than being governed by the fear of the shaming vulnerability of losing power. We long for people groups that have historically known nothing but enmity to peacefully create space for being known and leave the nuclear weapon of contempt outside the conversation.

But evil has other plans and uses shame as a primary emotional leverage not simply to entice humans to "do something wrong" or "disobey," although that certainly is what they did in the Genesis story, but to disrupt relationships via its access to functions of the mind that do not emerge from the parts of the brain that make us uniquely human. Rather, it activates systems within the brainstem and limbic circuitry that, given our penchant for inattentiveness, wreak havoc on our prefrontal cortices. It utilizes contempt, even in the mildest forms, to create patterns of distress in response to which we create coping strategies—idols—that forgo relationships for things we believe we can more independently control and that will pose less risk for hurting us in the future.

Unfortunately, this invariably leads to the isolation of hiding from ourselves, from each other and from God, continuing to make up our stories on our own, terrified of collaborating in the telling of stories with others for fear that our nakedness will be revealed and exploited. The eventual, inevitable outcome of this isolation is hell, the antithetical state of the we-ness and with-ness of life in trinitarian community. It is the counter echo of God's mandate that it is not good to be alone. Shame's power lies in its subtlety and silence, embedded in mental functions of implicit memory that we carry individually and corporately, and is quite content to remain in the shadows while we go on to do its dirty work. It extends and nourishes itself, devouring us in the process, as our individual shame mushrooms into its various corporate expressions. We remain in its self-perpetuating cycle of judgment and hiding, continuing to fulfill the prophecy of the curses that God has foreseen.

This is the beginning of our story as told by the Bible. For many of us this is the story we still live in. What are we to do?

The solution lies, ironically, in doing the very thing that shame convinces us is the most dangerous, threatening act we could commit. What a surprise to find that in the story we have just read, we already have the beginnings of what God intends to do to show us the way.

# 6

# Shame's Remedy: Vulnerability

The lying began long before the sex. But with the sex, the lying came more easily, more consciously—and necessarily. Carla had never intended for life to turn out like this. But she was unable to imagine changing course, certain that doing so would result in catastrophe for her marriage, her children, her work and her community. The only solace she seemed to find was in the arms of the ongoing affair.

She was referred to me because of her insomnia, and what she wanted was something to help her sleep. In her story, coming to see a psychiatrist was about finding a solution to a problem with her biorhythms. She was not expecting it to take such a sharp, right-angle turn.

"Tell me about your marriage," I said. Treating sleep disorders is certainly about biochemistry and brain function. It is no less about relationships. She replied, "My marriage is fine." As anyone who speaks with a mental health professional might know, when you use the word *fine* to describe anything, you're asking for the full-court exploratory press. She went on to discuss how staid and boring things had become with her husband, Preston. He seemed so passive and uninterested in her ever since their second child had been born. This inevitably led to more conversation about what she was doing with all her feelings about this seemingly most important relationship in her life.

With surprising nonchalance and candor she blurted out, "I'm having an affair with my boss." Instantly her demeanor changed. It was as if she had been waiting for months, years even, to say this to someone, but the moment the cat was out of the bag, she recoiled in revulsion from what she had just admitted. Not unlike the immediate relief one experiences from having an abscess lanced, only to be sickened by the appearance and nature of the pus pouring forth. Her embarrassment was immediate and palpable, and she could barely speak, let alone look at me. Tears began to flow. I attempted to gently move closer to the topic and her fragile heart. "I don't want to talk about that. That's not what I'm here for. I just need to get some sleep."

I offered that perhaps the reason she revealed her affair was because she in fact *did* want to talk about it, but that shame much preferred that the abscess continue to fester until she was in full-blown emotional and relational sepsis. The session ended with my prescribing something to help her sleep—but not without her agreeing to return to talk more about her story. Which she did.

Over the course of several weeks, Carla revealed a narrative in which she worked hard as a middle child to gain the attention of her parents, who were busy raising five children. She exhibited competence at just about everything—relationships, academics, even her fledgling faith—so she seemed to have little need for anyone to seek her out, to be curious about her inner life of insecurities and dreams. The potential downside to never having anything to do with trouble in your family is the possibility that your family never suspects that trouble ever has anything to do with you.

It was not until she began to explore her story in more detail that her deeply rooted shame was given a linguistic framework. Had she had words for it before the affair, she might have declared that she was exhausted from working so hard at being competent and making sure that people around her were getting along with each other, never mind that her feelings were consistently left unattended. As she reflected on all of her accomplishments, she stated that part of her was tempted to believe her "competence" was fraudulent. That it was all a lie. An untruth told to cover up her real self, which felt invisible and small.

Despite her intellect and social aplomb, she carried the sense that she was not enough for her husband (why, otherwise, would he not pursue her?), not enough for her parents (although she loved and respected them, their attention frequently seemed focused on her siblings, but rarely on her), and not enough for God (despite how deeply she still desired to follow Jesus, she translated God's felt absence as his disappointment in her). These were some of the lies she believed. Lies that she told herself, often without words.

Subtle and silent, this undercurrent of shame followed her to the law firm where she worked, and where she felt seen and heard in novel and exhilarating ways. With the promotions, challenges and attention from her boss, her capacity to silence the voice of shame with her gifts expanded. But when her children were born that capacity began to thin. With demands coming from all sides—from her children both physically and emotionally; from her husband, who felt expendable; and from work, where she found the most satisfaction in her life—she began to feel overwhelmed. And when overwhelmed, Carla, like the rest of us, turned to her strengths, which lay in working harder at making people happy, especially those who were more likely to provide immediate gratification in their responses. And the most prominent source of that gratification occupied the corner office down the hall from her at the firm.

*This will not get out of hand,* she told herself. *I can handle this. He is only interested in my work, and I love my work.* The lies became more entrenched and automatic. They became as much who she was as what she told herself. Before she knew it, working lunches turned into working dinners, which turned into intimate conversations usually reserved for spouses or the closest of girlfriends. Her boss, of course, was in a listless marriage, and he had no trouble revealing his one area of neediness to which Carla gravitated to supply the emotional solution, something she had learned well how to do in her middle-child occupancy. With each step closer to the abyss, her boss was sending a message she interpreted as, "You are beautiful. You are smart. You are funny. You are the answer to all my questions. You are what I need. You are . . . enough." What she did not hear was him saying more implicitly, "I need you to meet my needs. My needs are more important than you or your marriage or your children. My needs are really all that matter to me. Your needs matter to me as long as meeting them is a way for me to ultimately meet my needs. For you, as it turns out, are not as important as you might think." These were the words that were implied despite what she heard him say.

Sexual involvement was the predictable next stop on her train's journey, though it initially carried with it no small amount of shame and guilt. How to keep the secret safe from Preston, from her close friends, from her parents? So much energy expended maintaining the façade, Carla unaware of the presence of the shame attendant constantly reminding her that her life was a lie and that she was not and would not be enough. And it certainly would not be enough if she stopped the affair. The only solution she had for these noxious feelings was to turn her attention to the sensations, images and feelings of how unconditionally loved she felt by her employer. At some point not long before Carla and I first met, her husband became suspicious; upon his inquiry, she flatly denied to him any extramarital relationship. No wonder she hadn't been sleeping. Shame's perfect loop was complete.

"What do you feel when I suggest the possibility of telling Preston about the affair?" I asked. She was aghast. "I feel like throwing up." Indeed, in the moments that followed she complained of feeling lightheaded and nauseated. "There is no conceivable universe in which that is happening. He's already uninterested in me. Now he will hate me—no, worse than hate. I would be repulsive to him. And I should be, given what I've done. What's more, if I tell him, he will leave me and take the boys, which he would more than have the right to do."

After several sessions, Carla eventually came to a point of realization. "I think I know why I can't tell him, and it boils down to this. I feel too . . . vulnerable." There. She said it. She uttered what many of us might easily say is one of the most uncomfortable sensations that we know. To feel vulnerable is to feel, as did Eve and Adam after their fruit fest, naked and ashamed. For in the story of the world portrayed in the biblical narrative, shame is the tacit emotional payload that vulnerability carries. In our minds, to be vulnerable is to sense the potential for danger. But this danger is not perceived as being merely that of physical annihilation, limited to the functions of the brainstem and limbic circuitry. It is the even more consciously terrifying prospect of relational disintegration, which eventually leads to the prefrontal cortex telling us we are not enough and the specter of our being left as a result. To be vulnerable is to recognize that we are at the mercy of those whose intentions we cannot guarantee, and who can leave us alone.

Into this state of vulnerability I offered to Carla another way of picturing what was taking place in her interpersonal neurobiological matrix. "It makes complete sense that you would feel so vulnerable," I said. "This is the feeling that shame activates and that everyone feels to some degree when they are on the verge of being known in what they anticipate may be an unsafe space. To allow yourself to be known is very hard work." In the language of the Bible, vulnerability is reframed and transformed into something completely different. Something that only the story of the Bible—only the God of the Bible—can offer. As it does, it invites us to offer the same to each other. The gift—and the terror—of being known.

Carla could see that her anticipation of feeling intensely vulnerable—and the shame that was embedded within it—stood in the way of the movement she needed to make if her life was to be redeemed. She was surprised to discover that this sense of vulnerability, which she interpreted as the sign of her greatest weakness—the greatest risk to her survival—when reframed in terms of being known by (in this case) me, and hopefully God and perhaps even her husband, was in fact the key to her healing. But how was she to realize this? How was she to swim across this river of fire?

## Who We Are, Not Who We Wish to Be

We tend to think of vulnerability as something we experience at particular times or occasions. We sense it when we are criticized, when we are ill, when we have been fired from a job, when we have a difficult conversation with someone we perceive has more power than we do, when we have to speak in front of an audience or have to defend a dissertation. Or, in Carla's case, when we are about to reveal something that could potentially lead to painful consequences. Regardless of the occasion, we consider being exposed as something that happens at a distinct time and within the context of a particular event.

This is not an inaccurate description of what it means to feel vulnerable, but it is not complete. In reality, vulnerability is not something we choose or that is true in a given moment, while the rest of the time it is not. Rather, it is something we *are*. This is why we wear clothes, live in houses and have speed limits. So much of what we do in life is designed, among other things, to protect us from the fact that we are vulnerable *at all times*. To be human *is* to be vulnerable. In fact, it may be argued that no other animal, in its completely natural, naked state, is more vulnerable than we are. But we have more ways than do antelope for dealing with all the things that could otherwise remind us of that fact. Vulnerability is not a question of if but rather to what degree. This does not imply that we have no choices of being more openly so, but it is an illusion to believe that we are not vulnerable. It is something we can hide but not that we can eliminate. The question, then, is not *if* we are or will be vulnerable but rather *how* and *when* we enter into it consciously and intentionally for the sake of creating a world of goodness and beauty.

In the abstract, our constant vulnerability is not difficult to grasp. And there are many dimensions of how this presents itself. We are physically vulnerable, to be certain. No one can predict that he or she will be alive at the end of the day, given that we could be run over by a bus. But we have a fair amount of control over that. I can choose to stay off roads where buses operate. However, in our deeply interactive relational lives vulnerability becomes more tricky. We avoid physical vulnerability, which only makes sense, for it risks the ultimate danger of death. Since we make avoiding physical vulnerability a priority, being open to relational vulnerability cuts against the grain of all we have been programmed to do. Given that our minds are embodied, we should expect that when we practice something with our bodies our minds are molded into a similar form.

We so thoroughly guarantee our physical safety that we believe vulnerability is abnormal, even pathological. Certainly, we would never expect to see an advertisement that encourages vulnerability. Strength and fearlessness are expected and promoted by this world's dominant plausibility structure. Survival of the fittest is not easily translated into a dialect that includes vulnerability. Weakness, which is often equated with vulnerability, is not welcome. Given the myriad ways we protect our vulnerable selves, we eventually believe that we *are* not and *should* not be vulnerable. This is why our moments of emotional vulnerability are seen as episodic events that are not the norm. And they are often viewed as indicating that something is wrong. The various ways we both demonstrate vulnerability and protect ourselves against it has been helpfully described by Brené Brown.[1] That her work has been so well-received is a testimony to how universal the phenomenon of vulnerability is, yet how much energy we burn to avoid it.

For Carla, and for the rest of us, the idea of vulnerability brings with it both the hope of liberation and the terror of possible abject rejection. For those of us who see it as a weakness, it may be helpful—as it was for Carla—to be reminded of the story we believe we are living in.

## CREATED TO BE VULNERABLE

Like shame, vulnerability is understood to be an artifact of the human condition. The work of Brown and others has drawn the public's attention to its potential to enhance human flourishing.[2] This notwithstanding, from the standpoint of naturalistic evolution it merely functions as a moderator of human interactions. Although we may now be discovering its helpfulness, historically it has remained unrelated to any ultimate understanding within our larger story as human beings.

But the biblical narrative tells a different story. One so different, in fact, that in seeing the place of vulnerability in the pages of the Bible we cannot help but be amazed at its place and purpose. It begins in the beginning, where we are introduced to a vulnerable God. Vulnerable in the sense that he is open to wounding. Open to pain. Open to rejection. Open to death.

Like shame, recent sociological research about the place and function of vulnerability affirms what the biblical narrative has for over four millennia been telling us about humans and God. As we read about the triune God considering the possibility of creating humankind in his image (Genesis 1:26-27), we get the impression God knows that inviting humans to join him in this joyful life on earth would necessarily mean that God was setting himself up for a rough go of it. God put himself in harm's way simply by making us. The act of creation was one of vulnerability, an act in which God was open to wounding, with the anticipated heartache that accompanies it. However, this openness was bracketed by a relational connection that prevents fear and shame from ruling its anticipated future. Although we can assume that God knew creation would bring trouble, he had confidence that his triune relationships would bear the weight of whatever trauma would come his way.

Further along in the creation narrative we see how the man and woman's shameless nakedness (Genesis 2:25) is a reflection of trinitarian interdependence and joy, a mirror of what it meant to be made in God's image ("in *our* image"). For the man and woman to be naked and unashamed *was* to be vulnerable, *was* to be open to wounding. It emphasized that they, in their vulnerable need, were dependent on each other in order for life to flourish. For surely it is not good for humans to be alone (Genesis 2:18). Our vulnerability reminds us that deep relationship is the norm, not something we periodically require when we are in trouble or are lonely. And this neurobiology of "we" reflects God's intention for our created purpose from the beginning.[3]

But naked vulnerability is not merely a representation of our having been created to be in relationship. God desires us to live like he lives. Thus, to be created in God's image also refers to our having creative dominion within the world. And to be maximally creative also requires that we are vulnerable. This is not the message that we hear in most of our interactions while gathered around the office water cooler. We are pressured to do things well on our own. And to the degree that we cannot, shame is waiting for us. One could argue that the most powerful creative act of humans lies on the continuum between sexual intercourse and the birth of a baby. Nothing requires more physical vulnerability than this life-fashioning act. Nor can it be accomplished alone. And so we see that nakedness is not just about *need* but also the joy of creating together something we cannot create on our own. Vulnerability is not just a random state of neediness or openness to danger. It is built into the cosmic fabric of the world to provide the opportunity for discovery and creation, and for the emergence of beauty and goodness.

## COMING TO FIND US

In Genesis 3, while all hell is breaking loose God looks for the first couple. As we saw in chapter five, what was once naked, creative innocence had devolved into hidden, isolated judgment. For the couple, to be vulnerable now carried the risk of contempt, no longer the opportunity for bringing something into being that was greater than the sum of its originating parts. Into this space God came walking "in the cool of the day." "Where are you?" Even in their newly fierce independence, he sought them out. God's inquiry elicits further distancing, greater shame and deeper conviction that vulnerability is not what it's cracked up to be.

It is easy for this passage to draw our attention primarily to what Adam and Eve are feeling and how they are responding. But what was God feeling as he inquired, "Where are you?" What must it have been like to have known, to have felt the rejection from humans? It is not hard to read this story and immediately conclude that the humans were rejecting God—for indeed they were. It may take more work for us to imagine that God actually felt that rejection, and though it did not keep him from continuing to seek us out, we have no reason to doubt that that moment was the first of many moments that would culminate on Good Friday. Only when we see Jesus do we begin to get a picture of what God may have been experiencing when his vulnerability was first exposed.

Notice that from the beginning, when God comes, he asks questions. *He* is the one pursuing answers. "Where are you?" The question assumes vulnerability is in order. He is seeking naked creativity. He is asking us to be as vulnerable as he was in creating us in the first place. He is looking for us because he longs for us to be *with him* even as he is with us, for us to know his delight with us which is present at all times, even in the presence of other things he may simultaneously feel. He is not asking the couple their whereabouts to acquire their geographic location, nor simply information about the state of their souls. His question is a means of connecting. He is not inviting them into a place of vulnerability merely for vulnerability's sake. Rather, vulnerability is the state we must pass through in order to deepen our connection with God and others, given our condition. There is no other way.

In God's movement toward reconciliation, he envisions the process as something that we do together. He does not come initially telling us what to do. That requires no trust, no vulnerability on the part of either of us. He comes asking questions. Questions that genuinely seek interactive relationship. It is not a bait-and-switch operation in which God isn't so much asking a question as making a statement. In fact, from the beginning God has had to trust us as much as he asks us to trust him. In creating us he risks everything—short of his trinitarian relational connection—something we often have great difficulty imagining. In the story we tell as followers of Jesus, then, from its opening pages we find vulnerability—first without shame and then in the face of it—to be an essential aspect of God's posture toward us and nothing short of a fundamental necessity for the healing of shame and the promotion of human flourishing.

But we must not forget that in the Christian narrative God's vulnerability hinges on something hinted at that is not yet fully developed in the pages of Genesis—but the seed of which is plainly present. It took generations of hard work, prayer and reflection for the doctrine of the Trinity to be established, which assents that the God of the Bible is a God of unity yet separate and distinct in his three persons. This is not the place to fully explore this mystery, but it is deeply important in addressing the problem of shame. As noted earlier, one of shame's most prominent features, and one that provides the emotional fuel of terror at the prospect of living vulnerably, is the threat of isolation, of abandonment. Our brains are wired with a deep suspicion of anything that might leave us alone in the ultimate sense. Thus, we are reluctant to expose ourselves, fearful that in so doing we may, once connected, be left. For indeed, we see even in Genesis that if we trust ourselves to vulnerability, bad things can eventually happen. It was only in the state of nakedness that Adam and Eve opened themselves to what they did to each other. The more of me that is exposed to another, the greater will be my wounding when I am betrayed. We deeply long for connection, to be seen and known for who we are without rejection. But we are terrified of the vulnerability that is required for that very contact. And shame is the variable that mediates that fear of rejection in the face of vulnerability.

But in the Trinity we see something that we must pay attention to: God does not leave. The loving relationship shared between Father, Son and Spirit is the ground on which all other models of life and creativity rest. In this relationship of constant self-giving, vulnerable and joyful love, shame has no oxygen to breathe. The ever-present movement of this three-part, shared relationship toward one another—working with one another, trusting one another, delighting in one another—provides the basis for why God created the world in vulnerability, and then made himself vulnerable in coming to it in Jesus.

This imaged trinitarian relationship is where all healing begins for followers of Jesus. And for Carla and countless others like her, this relationship invited her into the beginning of vulnerability and the end of her shame. Needless to say, none of this was easy. Fortunately, she discovered that God knows exactly what that is like.

## COMING TO BE KNOWN

Carla indeed was being invited into relationship. In the moments in my office when she felt vulnerable, she was actually on the verge of something that the Bible frames very differently. In *Anatomy of the Soul* I explored what it means to *be known*.[4] St. Paul refers to this in 1 Corinthians 8:2-3, where he points out the difference between knowing in order to master the universe and being known by God: "Those who think they know something do not yet know as they ought to know. But whoever loves God is known by God."

Paul indicates that being known by God is the signpost that we love him. And to be known necessarily means that we are willing to expose each part of us, especially those parts that feel most hidden and that carry the most shame. For to *know* as in verse 2 is not unlike what Adam and Eve sought in the fruit of the tree of knowledge of good and evil. It is to ask all the questions and do all the observing and analyzing. In contrast, to *be known* is necessarily to be vulnerable, to open ourselves to God's love. It is to be asked questions. To be observed. To be seen.

And as David Benner points out, those parts of us that feel most broken and that we keep most hidden are the parts that most desperately

need to be known by God, so as to be loved and healed.[5] These are the
parts that contain our shame. And our shame attendant incessantly
draws our attention to them. God came to find Eve and Adam to provide
them the opportunity to be known as he knows anything else. For only
in those instances when our shamed parts are known do they stand a
chance to be redeemed. We can love God, love ourselves or love others
only to the degree that we are known by God and known by others. Carla
was beginning that journey, and it was not proving to be easy.

These parts will know the greatest joy in healing as they are known. In
1 Corinthians 13:12, Paul, writing in the poetic language of a hymn, reminds us that "now we see only a reflection as in a mirror; then we shall
see face to face. Now I know in part; then I shall know fully, even as I am
fully known."

To be fully loved—and to fully love—requires that we are fully known.
Absolute joy comes not just in my having some random joyful engagement with something or someone. Rather, absolute joy must eventually include my being completely known, especially those parts that in
subtle, hidden ways have carried shame, often without my conscious
awareness. This is the language of the new heaven and new earth. This is
the work that God alone has initiated and in which he longs for us to join
him. For God longs to be known by us as much as he longs for us to be
known by him. He desires us to join him in his trinitarian life of being
known. It is not unreasonable to suggest that in Eden God was as interested in a conversation, real engagement, as much as he was interested
in pointing out what the man and the woman had done wrong. He was
more eager to be known and for them to be known than he was for them
to be shamed. This has not changed. To the degree that we practice being
known in this age, we will be that much more ready for its full expression
in the age to come. But again, this requires work unsurpassed in difficulty by any other human undertaking.

The imagery of the Bible's story of vulnerability is set apart from the
world's story in that the biblical narrative tells of a God who is with us in
this process of exposure. In the midst of vulnerability, shame colors our
sense of it in such a way that we feel quite alone. To be known presumes

that we are not in isolation but that there is *another* by whom and in whose willing and eager presence we are being known. In the story centered around Jesus we read "Come to me all you who are weary and burdened, and I will give you rest" (Matthew 11:28), and "Come near to God and he will come near to you" (James 4:8). The moment we are conscious of feeling vulnerable, we have activated our sense of being alone. But as he did when seeking Adam and Eve, God invites us to live as we were made to live—in relationship, *with* him and *with* others, in the state of being known, not in the state of isolation that shame desires.

## COMING TO STAY

In the Genesis account, and for much of the Old Testament, we are told a story of a God of movement. A God who comes and goes, yet who tells us that he never leaves us alone. A God who longs for us to be known by him and who longs to be known by us. We must learn this same lesson developmentally. As newborns and infants we need the presence of our parents virtually at all times. But over time we learn that they can also come and go, but remain "with us" in our minds, as our memory capacity begins to mature.

But we don't learn that lesson as easily when it comes to God. We have a hard time believing, living as if, we are in his mind. And we have difficulty keeping him in ours. Perhaps this is why Isaiah 7–8 hints at what we eventually read in the Matthew 1. For in both of these texts we read of Immanuel. We hear of a God who comes to pitch his tent among ours. A God who in Jesus is not merely with us as a chair is with us, but who sees us, speaks with us, sits at our table for a meal and asks us questions. Questions that require of us great vulnerability, none of which he asks privately but rather before others: "What do you want me to do for you?" (Mark 10:51). "Do you want to get well?" he continues (John 5:6). "Who do you say I am?" Jesus asked of his disciples (Mark 8:29).

But he not only asks questions. In addition to telling us how to live ("I tell you, love your enemies and pray for those who persecute you" [Matthew 5:44]), he revealed himself to us in exceedingly vulnerable ways: "I and the Father are one" (John 10:30); "I am the bread of life" (John 6:35);

"I am the light of the world" (John 8:12). It is easy for us to hear these as words of comfort and calling. But what did it mean to Jesus to say them? What emotion coursed through him as he revealed these deeply intimate parts of who he saw himself to be? These words were not mere declarations of truth. They were acts of vulnerability, for in his context he opened the door to ridicule, rejection and eventual subjection to torturous death.

There is no indication that he made these declarations naively. Nor that he was a paragon of supremely confident impregnibility, fearless throughout his progression from Bethlehem to Golgotha. Rather, that he was enveloped in the relationship revealed at his baptism and heard in the words "You are my Son, whom I love; with you I am well pleased" (Luke 3:22). Indeed, in his wrestling with Satan in the desert immediately following his baptism and just prior to his ministry's commencement (Matthew 4:1-11; Mark 1:9-13; Luke 4:1-13), he addressed imagined escape routes from the path he eventually took, Teflon-paved routes of invulnerability that would have avoided the mess that otherwise awaited him.

Likewise, at the conclusion of his ministry, Jesus finds himself in Gethsemane pleading with his father to remove "this cup," which perhaps represented not just crucifixion but all that he would take upon himself—sin—our refusal of relationship, our turning away from love and our commitment to making our way in the world by ourselves. And the shame of the cross would herald, promote and reinforce sin, becoming inextricably intertwined with it. Jesus' crucifixion is as emblematic of shame as it is of sin. Crucifixion was intended not only to execute victims but to simultaneously humiliate them.

Before being crucified, victims were usually stripped naked. It is difficult to imagine a more humiliating event. There is reason to believe this was true for Jesus. But we find it virtually impossible to look upon his naked form, or even consider it, given how embarrassing it feels. Our own discomfort is revealed even in the way we represent it artistically. With few exceptions, depictions of this event usually portray Jesus' loins covered with a cloth. This is not to argue in favor of a different way to portray Jesus' crucifixion, but rather to point out that although we assent theologically to how Good Friday delivered us from shame as well as sin, actually permitting ourselves to be there on that Friday, being with a naked Jesus, is an entirely different matter altogether. But only to the degree that we take the time to image, sense and feel what it would have been like to be there can we answer yes to the question "Were you there when they crucified my Lord?"

The point here is to emphasize that Jesus' literal naked vulnerability is a testimony to us that *he knows exactly what it is like to be us.* To truly be with us Jesus—Immanuel—not only knows what it means to be vulnerable, he knows how painfully, frighteningly hard it is to live into it, given shame's threat. He knows the agony of sweating blood, looking for a way—any way—to avoid being stripped naked, being seen for who he was and left alone to die. He does not require anything of us that he does not first do himself. When the time came for Carla to consider coming clean about her affair—and about her lifelong striving to be seen, to be heard, to be enough—I mentioned that I imagined Jesus, far from looking at her with impatience, might more likely tell her that he knows, despite its necessity, just how painfully hard it is to expose herself, given shame's power.

To *this* God, whom we meet in Jesus, we must direct our attention if we are to know the healing of our shame. We must literally look to Jesus in embodied ways in order to know how being loved in community brings shame to its knees and lifts us up and into acts of goodness and beauty. To this God Carla began to nudge closer, desperate to find breath as she anticipated what she feared to be her certain, impending drowning.

## THE DEVIL'S IN THE (SMALLEST) DETAILS

With Carla's story it is tempting to be distracted into imagining that shame is only sensed, imaged, felt, thought about or acted on in dramatically tragic or sensational settings. In Carla's narrative its presence and nature are patently obvious; the intensity of the vulnerability she felt as she considered confessing the truth to her husband is no less comprehensible. Likewise, it takes little effort to acknowledge Jesus' vulnerability and the reality of shame's attempt to literally strip him into a state of disintegration. But we must be wise, for shame would like nothing more than for us to believe that it only shows up in grand style, that it only speaks when we hear it loudest in the most glaring situations. In considering Carla's story, it would be easy for us to assume that shame—serious shame—is mostly about her affair. But we would be wrong.

Carla's life is an example of how shame's tactics work. It begets itself. Again, we must be careful not to assume that shame became visible and active only when she entered her affair. But the affair was in many respects the *result* of shame as much as it was its cause. This is how it tends to work. We don't find ourselves shaming others loudly in the staff meeting apart from our own shame telling us that we are not enough. We do not embezzle unless at some deep level we believe we are not enough without the money. We continually look at pornography in no small part as a coping mechanism for our inadequacy that long precedes it. We don't avoid hard conversations in our marriages without our conviction that we don't have what it takes to tolerate what will inevitably be said, which will lead to someone leaving, someone living out in words or actions that we are not enough. In all these and hundreds of other seemingly innocuous moments, shame begins with a whisper and crescendos to a roar, as it did with Carla.

Shame, as it turns out, lives in the smallest of details, the commonest of life's moments, and that is exactly where it wants to remain. Yes, it comes into the bedroom of a child, the victim of her grandfather's sexual abuse; there are few screenplays more ugly and tragic than this. More often, however, it lives in the less obvious glance or tone of voice that lasts but a second and lingers for weeks. It thrives in the silence of questions of genuine curiosity never asked, words of encouragement or thanks or praise never offered. It emerges in the emotional neglect that seems so minor until its accumulated absence leaves that neglected child with no option but to imagine a story, mostly as a silent movie, in which he is not important to his father. And this will seep into the story he tells himself about what it means for him to be a friend, a sibling, a husband and a father himself. But it will also infect what he senses who he is to God. Shame loves to tell its version of a good tale.

It sits in boardrooms where the directors, fearing the shame that fuels their own vulnerability, refuse to make the hard choices necessary to effectively care for their employees, while continuing to permit the CEO to behave irresponsibly. It walks in school hallways and into classrooms where administrators, fearing funding cuts, drive their teachers, who drive their students, who drive their parents crazy, who in their fear of not being enough, complain that the administrators are not doing enough to get their children into Yale. It lurks in the academy where if a professor does not produce, she is not noticed, and if not noticed tenure won't be realized. And the backbiting and gossip and undermining—the noble commitment to the pursuit of knowledge notwithstanding—become an accepted part of life in the department at the university. Shame is in the words of our sermons and our Facebook posts about those sermons. It is in our rhetoric about sexuality and immigration. Shame screams at players on the court and at soldiers in basic training. It writes and speaks about the politician as well as her opponent, depending on which paper's editor has the pen. It repeatedly tells a story of the world that is made up of "we" and "they." And "they" are always the bad guys. And the bad guys always end up on the open end of the barrel of a gun. Judgment, as it turns out, comes easily in the form of fiery words or hot lead. Both leave bodies on the field with no one to tend the wounded. Shame, as we know, is no respecter of persons; we who follow Jesus often find that we have as much difficulty with this as anyone, I being the chief among sinners.

And we have become numb to this, indifferently resigned, unconsciously conceding, "This is the way life is." And the way of life is the way of shame. Shame, as evil's vector would like it to be, keeps itself hidden among life's everyday events. It wants to be known merely as an artifact, something that we dislike intensely and would work to change, but that has no fundamental purpose. However, it intends to dismantle a world that was destined for goodness and beauty.

Who would risk imagining a story whose intended consummation is in a city whose tree bears the leaves that will be healing for the nations? Who would be crazy enough to believe there is a place where you can be naked and unashamed? Who would intentionally turn the focus of their attention toward shame in order to choke it to death? In what world could that scenario possibly exist?

Does the biblical notion of being known hold any hope to answer these questions? We have seen how it means that we, in the safety of a trusting relationship, expose our real selves, the parts of us that we perceive to be shameful, in small or large degree. We have also witnessed that God does not ask us to do anything he is not willing to do himself. And in Jesus, he has come to us, revealing himself to us for all that he is.

So we once again turn to interpersonal neurobiology—part of God's good creation—comprehending it through the plausibility structure of the biblical narrative. In so doing we will see how being known as God would have it heals our shame by drawing our attention to the story that Jesus both occupied and paid attention to himself. It is a story in which Jesus looked forward to the joy that will come in the presence of a great cloud of witnesses gathered around the throne of God. This process of being known opens the door not only for healing but for the expansion of our capacity to co-create with God renewed minds and hearts, out of which burst a kingdom of goodness and beauty in the face of shame's withering onslaught.

# 7

# Our Healing Cloud of Witnesses

For Carla, telling me about the affair was just the beginning. The felt risk continued to mount as she moved eventually to telling a trusted friend, then her pastor, then finally revealing her story to her husband while both of them were in my office. Carla and Preston's story is one of painful recovery and a marriage not only saved but now thriving. Not all stories end so well. Nor have they easily forgotten their past. And shame has tried to make a valiant comeback along the way. But their journey out of their shame and into a life of flourishing joy was realized not least because of their willingness to be known. It is not difficult to suggest, therefore, that the process of being known is necessary for the healing of shame. But what practical steps do we take to address the mind-body state of shame, given that it so thoroughly infects and disintegrates every functional domain of the mind? How do we confront it, given that it is highly resistant to efforts that are often limited to changing what we think rationally? In addition to revealing the truth about their marriage, indeed their whole lives, Carla and Preston were able to diminish the influence of shame in a concrete way by practicing the very thing that intuitively we are prone to avoid.

## WATCH WHAT HE DOES, DO WHAT HE DOES
In the New Testament letter to the Hebrews, we are provided with a model for how to effectively approach our nemesis:

> Therefore, since we are surrounded by such a great cloud of witnesses, let us throw off everything that hinders and the sin that so easily entangles. And let us run with perseverance the race marked out for us, fixing our eyes on Jesus, the pioneer and perfecter of faith. For the joy set before him he endured the cross, scorning its shame, and sat down at the right hand of the throne of God. (Hebrews 12:1-2)

The imagery of a "great cloud of witnesses" refers to those just named in chapter 11 (those that have gone before us) and to those who are with us now, emphasizing that we are not alone on our journey.

It requires great effort, however, to keep before us this vision of being part of a great gathering of people cheering us on, telling us "Well done!" as we move through life. This is one of the first and most helpful steps in combating shame. It entails creating communities around us who are reminding us of the same thing that Jesus heard at his baptism. Our struggle against shame is begun not by ourselves but in the company of trustworthy friends, family members and spiritual mentors. Remember, isolation is one of shame's primary methods. We therefore must be cautious of thinking that we can do this by ourselves through sheer force of will.

Next, the writer of the text invites us to put aside everything that holds us back from running the race with perseverance. The phrase "the sin that so easily entangles" is translated by other ancient authorities as the sin that so easily "distracts." This is helpful because so much sin begins as a function of attention. Shame functions first, as Satan did with Eve, by drawing our attention, even in minute moments, away from our focus on God's voice telling us that we are loved and that he is pleased with us, along with the necessary sensations, images and feelings that accompany it. Remember, attention is the key to the engine that pulls the train of our mind; shame's first priority is distraction.

We then read that we are to fix our eyes—our attention—on Jesus. Essentially we are called to watch and do what he does, to follow his example. In *Anatomy of the Soul* I describe Jesus' experience of hearing his Father telling him, "You are my son, whom I love; with you I am well pleased," which is what God is telling all of his sons and daughters at all times (not to the exclusion of other things he is also saying). What set Jesus apart was that he heard it and acted on it. It is imperative that we do the same. Shame will do everything it can to distract us from this message. Jesus knew this and took measures to excise those parts of his own life that shame would attempt to exploit as he began his ministry.

Immediately following his baptism, Jesus "was led by the Spirit into the wilderness" (Luke 4). You have heard the saying that it is wise to keep our friends close and our enemies closer. Jesus knew he needed to closely engage Satan in order to recognize when shame was in play. In all three instances of temptation, Jesus confronted the parts of his mind that evil tried to use to distract him. "If you are the Son of God, turn these stones into bread. . . . Jump off the temple. . . . Commit to my style of running the world politically through force." In each case, Satan questions God's pleasure with Jesus. "Look, if God really loved you that much, why would he make it this hard? You have all these gifts. Use them! Or is it possible that God really doesn't love you in the way you think he does? Perhaps *Son* is a bit too strong to be using to describe yourself." Satan wants to convey that what Jesus planned to do was not going to be enough (thus the other options), that Jesus was not enough. "That being true, how could you possibly be God's Son? How could he possibly be pleased with you? Well, perhaps he is not." Echoes of a conversation long ago in Eden abound.

But Jesus counters this by saying over and over, "It is written . . ." This was not some primitive cognitive therapeutic technique, some ritual or mental talisman that he used to ward off intrusive thoughts. For any first-century Jew, what "is written" is shorthand for "God says." It is the tagline that draws Jesus' attention (there's that word again) to God's voice. Everything he reminds himself of pays attention to his relationship with his Father who loves him, is pleased with him, will be faithful to meet his deepest longings and will bring Jesus' creative calling to its climax. As he listens to his Father's voice reminding him who he is, Jesus remains intimately connected to his Father. At the end of Jesus' temptations in the desert, the Gospel writer reports that the devil left Jesus "for another time." This informs us that Jesus' journey into the wilderness was not a one-time trial. However, it prepared him for how shame would show up later in evil's attempt to convince Jesus that he was not God's Son, that he was not enough.

## PRACTICING ACTS OF IMAGINATION

To "fix our eyes on Jesus" means watching him and doing what he did. It is to intentionally seek out our shame, expose it and reframe it in light of our Father telling us that we are his daughters and sons in whom he is well-pleased. For this to happen, we must practice embodied acts of imagination that enable all our sensations, images, feelings, thoughts and physical actions to reflect our sense of God's delight with us.

What constitutes embodied acts of imagination? First, it includes fostering relationships that facilitate our hearing more distinctly our Father's voice of delight. Concretely, this means regularly and intentionally revealing our most hidden shame in the context of those relationships that comprise the great cloud of witnesses surrounding us. In this literal embodied act, our whole self is liberated from shame.

When I see my friend's face, hear his voice, sense his empathy for my plight in real time and space, I am given the opportunity to imagine a different way of telling the story of what has been only shame, isolation and stasis. To imagine a different story requires my brain to be in a position to do so; for I cannot imagine a future if I have no memory on which to base it. Embodied acts of this kind provide the basis for imagining new possibilities. But this takes effort and perseverance.

In my own life, I have been the beneficiary of several relationships in which I have practiced telling the truth about my deepest shameful secrets (and believe me, I have plenty). *Practice* is a crucial word, for I am quite imperfect at this discipline. Sometimes I easily look for ways to avoid acknowledging those shameful things that entangle me, distracting me from God's voice of delight. However, though we are imperfect, we are not necessarily ineffective.

For both Carla and Preston it was important to practice these acts of imagination and to immerse themselves in experiences that reinforced their conviction that they were loved and that their shame was to be dismissed. This required more than just marriage therapy. It required connection to other communities whose mission was to strengthen their memory of joy and forgiveness, while calling them to new life as individuals as well as a couple. They worked on this by joining a couples' group who met regularly and were committed to the mission of being fully known. In this place they both told their story. And over time, in this embodied community, they received the empathy they needed to risk trusting a newly imagined story, one of healing, redemption and joy. As that community frequently told this new story, Carla and Preston began to live it. Out of this Carla and Preston realized not only a way to forgive the past but also to create a new future in which they more vigilantly knew the place where shame would attempt to disrupt and disintegrate their relationship.

Significantly, when one member of a group formed with the intention of providing a context for healing risks revealing the vulnerable, broken and especially shameful parts of his or her story, a number of interpersonal neurobiological events are put in motion. First, it takes great courage to share something shameful (especially if the person has done something he or she is guilty of and feels shame as a matter of course). We see it in the person's face and body language—we have all been there. But almost immediately, we also witness a visible softening in the listeners' bodies: leaning forward in their seats toward the speaker, looks of compassion on their faces, kindness in their voices as they respond. As they do so, the speaker's own neurophysiologic state begins to change, as his or her brain feels felt by others. This initiates a greater level of neural network integration within the speaker, and with this comes less anxiety. Furthermore, having taken this risk, the person feels less alone in the story, for telling it now includes awareness of others' emotional acceptance of what is being felt. This is not to be equated with acceptance of bad behavior, merely the validation of the feeling that accompanies it.

With practice of such interactions, the speaker collects a new set of memories of what it means to live vulnerably with others. He or she begins to live not only as if "I will be okay" in the future when taking this kind of risk, but also lives in the present moment as if "I *am* okay." The speaker has the opportunity to grow in resilience as he or she learns how to loosen shame's grip on life by living transparently as often as possible. This type of community provides one way for its members to practice vulnerability and strengthen their ability to make this a way of life in all other relational contexts they inhabit.

The listeners in these groups are not merely empathically feeling something on behalf of the speaker, their role being limited to that of sounding boards, but they also are responding to what they are sensing *within themselves about their own story*, even without their knowing it at first. In this way we see how telling the truth about our lives—movement in and of itself—begets movement in those who are listening, evokes curiosity and consideration in others about their own brokenness, helping others to knit together different functional parts of their minds and helping them to make sense of things that heretofore have eluded them. This movement is terminally threatening to shame.

With practice listeners become aware that their responses to the speaker are as much about them as they are about the speaker. This is what being known in this way does: it moves people to greater places of connection to and greater integration with one another while each member simultaneously experiences enhanced integration within his or her own mind. Hence, when shame is being exposed and healed in the person revealing it, God simultaneously makes possible the healing of shame for all persons intimately participating in that person's story-telling effort.

Carl Rogers and Henri Nouwen have said that those things that are most personal are most universal. There is no greater evidence for this than when someone reveals the shame he or she carries while gathered in a group of safe, expectant listeners. I have said elsewhere that we all are born into the world looking for someone looking for us, and that we remain in this mode of searching for the rest of our lives. When we acknowledge our shame, it resonates with the shame carried by all of us. With confession, it is given the opportunity for resonance, exposure and healing in the life of the listener as well as the speaker. True goodness and beauty emerge when healing takes place at all levels of human awareness, which necessarily includes our individual as well as communal life. They are inseparable. This is what it means to be made in God's image. And this is what it means for us to live like God: to practice asking questions, the mission being not to find the right answers, important as they are, so much as to be more connected.

## TAKING INVENTORY OF SHAME

Next in Hebrews 12 we see that Jesus endured the cross, "scorning its shame." Other translations offer "disregarding" or "despising" for the word *scorning*. All of these words refer to an intentional act rather than being reactive. If we attended a party that our enemy also attended, but we eventually left without knowing that person was present, it could not be said that we scorned or disregarded our enemy at the party. Rather, to scorn, disregard or despise something, we must be aware of its presence. This is what Jesus did—and does—with shame. He seeks it out and does not blink in its presence. He does not pretend it is not there. In the end he did not shy away from crucifixion but approached it head-on, and then scorned, disregarded, despised the shame that it represented. By engaging his vocation, he accepted the shame that was necessarily part of it, shame that up to the moment of his death still tried to coax him into another way. We read that he was invited to come down from the cross and prove that he really was the Son of God (Mark 15:30); and in Matthew 26:53 Jesus reflected that he could call twelve legions of angels to his assistance.

In order to do what Jesus did requires that we seek shame where it hides. We do not wait for it to find us. An exercise I frequently use is called the shame inventory. It is a simple exercise using a 3 x 5 card and a pencil. Throughout the day, any time you encounter shame, make a mark on the card. The purpose is not to analyze what led to the shame or the larger story surrounding it. That form of analyzing, ironically, tends to feed the shame cycle. The purpose is to draw your attention to the fact that it has occurred. Remember, shame uses clandestine operations. It would be happy for you to experience it without it taking any credit. Its objective is not to be famous but to destroy you.

Remember that shame shows up in multiple mental functions: sensations, images, feelings, thoughts and behaviors. The goal of this exercise is to become increasingly aware of shame's activity as it presents itself in these various ways beyond "the voices I hear in my head" (although they are a common culprit). You are essentially becoming more proficient tracking the work of your shame attendant.

Usually, our responses to shame are so unconscious and automatic that we continue down that particular neurobiological path without realizing we are caught in shame's web until bad things are happening. This is what happened to Carla. But the very act of recognizing shame means that we stop and shift our attention in such a way that we interrupt our progression down the shame trail. In so doing, we give ourselves the opportunity to chart a different course.

For example, months after her confession, as Carla and Preston worked to rebuild their marriage, Carla reported that whenever she sensed Preston to be distant, she was overrun by images and feelings of her former boss, along with a sinking sensation in her chest, accompanied by the thought *I wish I weren't in this marriage.* This was soon followed with the self-judging thought *I made such a mistake!* All of this occurred in less than three seconds. It was not just words of accusation that she thought; it was the full complement of the mind's functional domains being assaulted by shame's attack.

Needless to say, this easily led to intensification of her feelings, which at times would lead to a souring of their interactions over the course of the entire afternoon and evening. By beginning to practice interrupting this initial image-feeling-thought complex and by naming it as a shame assault, Carla was able to put distance between the experience and her sense of herself, take a step back and begin again from where she was, which included telling Preston that she felt distance between them and she wanted to be closer. In so doing, she evoked in Preston the response of desiring to be closer, rather than feeling criticized for having been "distant." This continued to build confidence in their relationship, because prior to her confession he easily doubted her desire for closeness with him. This is an example of how intentionally acknowledging that shame was attempting to disintegrate the moment led to their becoming more deeply connected. This was not the story that shame planned on telling. Rather, it was the story of redemption, the story of God's kingdom breaking into the world in real time and space, the story that God wants to tell every moment of every day in each of our lives. If only we have ears to hear it and voices to tell it.

We often say in psychotherapy that we name things to tame things. Simply naming the moment as a shame event shifts our attention, taking us out of its vortex, allowing us to observe it more dispassionately and preventing us from unwittingly and automatically acting out of our Hebbian networks only to reinforce shame's message. What both Carla and Preston discovered, however, was that conducting the shame inventory became a part-time job—but only for a limited period of time—given how many times they noted shame's activity in the course of their day. As I reminded them, the purpose of the exercise is not to further shame us by reminding us how often shame is active in our life; rather it is to increase our awareness of shame in order to practice not permitting it to go any further once we have discovered and named it.

## SCORNING SHAME, PERSEVERING IN GOD'S STORY

The next step in this process involves shifting our attention from shame—and the story it is trying to tell—back to the story that is true, the story that God is telling in this very moment. To scorn or disregard shame is to acknowledge it and turn away, as if we think nothing of it.

This process of seeking shame to reveal where it hides so we may scorn it is made possible by our ongoing interactions with others who know us deeply. The image of Jesus' Spirit-mediated relationship with his Father models what this is to be. But Jesus also demonstrated for us how God pursues us to enable us to fearlessly confront our own shame while not being overrun by it, as his reinstatement of Peter demonstrates in John 21:15-17.[1] This interaction offers us a glimpse of how Jesus ferrets out Peter's shame and reorients his attention toward Jesus and to the work that Jesus was calling him to do. This is essentially how the practice of disregarding or scorning shame works. Eventually we are enabled to do this on a regular basis throughout our day, but only via the rhythmic reconnection with others to whom we faithfully confess the truth of our lives, not least being the shame that we otherwise are tempted to hide. We recall that stasis is one of shame's neurobiological attributes. It moves us literally and emotionally to places of isolation and paralysis. When we make a regular practice of sharing our lives with each other, we *move* toward them and create space for them to move toward us. Shame hates this.

Revealing our lives requires great perseverance. Returning to Hebrews 12:1, the writer flatly admonishes us to "run with perseverance the race marked out for us." We will not be rid of shame this side of the new heaven and earth; rather, we grow in our awareness of shame in order to scorn it. But we live in a world that speaks in the language of "fixing" things, of "mastering" problems. Shame would love for us to believe that we could be shame free; because when we find that we are not, we will be tempted once again to feel shame for still being tainted with it.

It is important for us to remind each other and ourselves that putting shame to death, as in crucifixion, is a slow process, and we are partnering with God as its executioners. Our mission is to continue in relationships that are arenas of light and safety in which confession of those parts of us where shame lurks becomes the norm. This will require great effort over time, for evil has no intention of going quietly into the night, though eventually it will indeed go. And as long as it has breath, it will have no more useful weapon at its disposal than shame. But with perseverance, we become more confident in confession as our means of creating space for God to bring us to greater places of integration and resilience, indeed for God to create within us undivided hearts.

Not only will we experience those benefits, but Hebrews 12:2 says, "For the joy set before him [Jesus] endured the cross, scorning its shame, and sat down at the right hand of the throne of God." The first thing we see, again, is joy. This is a recapitulation of creation. Joy was and is at the heart of God's trinitarian existence. For Jesus, "enduring the cross" is possible because before anything else, he is paying attention to the joy of being together with us in relationship with his Father in the Spirit. Joy is the byproduct of integration, of connection within a matrix of safe relationships. These relationships also place demands on us because they expect and hope that we will live in such a way so as to promote goodness and beauty. Joy, in this sense, is the outcome of Jesus' awareness of his Father's absolute delight in him, his joy in Jesus' presence, not just Jesus' behavior. Furthermore, this joy culminates in Jesus' eventual movement to carry out the vision for his place in the world: to be its Lord. In the same way, as we turn our attention to our Father's delight and do those things that facilitate our belief that this is the story we live in, we further create the proper space to discover domains of creativity, "good works, which God prepared in advance for us to do" (Ephesians 2:10).

For Preston and Carla, with the practice involved in being known by others—and others were known by them—joy began to emerge. At first it came only in the briefest moments of empathy, which could be easily missed and forgotten. But I and others brought their attention to those initial moments so they would remember them. And from those fragile memories joy sprung with even deeper resilience, in smiles and then laughter as they worked to fashion a reconstructed story out of the rubble of what had been. All of this happened in the context of being with other people who, themselves on a similar journey of redemption, joyfully welcomed Carla and Preston into their communities, shame and all.

## You're Right, You're Wrong

In chapter three I briefly mentioned that guilt stands on the platform of shame. We experience these as different albeit closely related affects. But I have never encountered someone who feels guilt without the under-current of shame to accompany and color it. For indeed, when our behavior causes relational ruptures—actions for which we are truly guilty, including those private actions of the mind that others may not immediately be aware of—our brain will sound the alarm, if even ever so faintly, of the injury of relational distancing. Shame, then, is as often related to our own wounding behavior toward others and ourselves as it is about the traumas we have sustained. It is, as it was for Eve, an indicator, a warning signal that one is relationally at risk.

It is significant, then, that as we listen to someone expressing shame associated with truly wrong behavior that we not turn a blind eye to such real relational breaches, or, in the language of the biblical narrative, to sin. The confession of shame is not a shortcut for hard work, some easy way to being let off the hook. In John 21 Jesus did not ignore Peter's denials. He did not minimize the depth of the wound Peter inflicted. And like Peter, we need to take responsibility for our actions that prove to be disintegrating. Not because God wants us to grovel or rub our noses in our brokenness, but that we learn and grow in our awareness of just how important our lives and connections to others really are. Again, we take the significance of our relationships far less seriously than God does.

When we wound others, creating either minor or gaping ruptures, it is necessary to repair them. This requires the admission of responsibility for our role in the rupture. Shame is the emotional energy behind our resistance to this. It does so by fueling our anticipation of being forsaken upon our admission of guilt. As we recall, one of shame's features is as a harbinger of abandonment, of catastrophic collapse of relationship. Even in small doses, when my left brain knows that my wife is not going to leave me when I admit to her that I have not done something I promised I would do, there still is the faint fear that redounds from hell. Lurking deep within us is what Satan convinced our first parents to believe—that we are not important enough for God to remain with us. Who looks forward to and enjoys the prospect of confessing to anyone a wrong committed? We might be able to imagine the relief in the absolution of guilt, but this requires that we work past shame's penchant for questioning whether we will be scorned rather than forgiven.

It is equally true that in order for me to be liberated from the shame I carry, I need someone to be able to say to me, "You're right. You were wrong to have done this." I need to hear that my behavior was *really as bad as I think, if not worse, while simultaneously sensing that the person I am confessing to is not leaving.* Shame has the effect of coaxing us into pretending that sin is not as bad it seems; for if it really is that bad, and I have to face it, it would be too much and I fear I would be overwhelmed. When someone seeks forgiveness for the wrong they have committed, we who have been wounded must be able to acknowledge the reality of the pain inflicted if forgiveness is to be real, and if the offender's shame is to be effectively healed.

For Carla and Preston, it took months before the sting of the shame of her affair lessened to tolerable levels. And it did, but not without Preston regularly revisiting her actions and practicing forgiveness, and Carla just as frequently accepting it, practicing the scorning of shame in order to reimagine her marriage in light of the story God was trying to tell rather than the one evil was fully committed to telling.

## THE POWER OF HEALING COMMUNITIES

From these reflections we can see how God can use a committed group of people to corporately make space to create undivided hearts, scorning shame and pushing it to the margins of our lives. To put shame to death requires being part of such a community. However, our nature is to live as if we can do everything on our own, and indeed that notion comes from the heart of evil itself. We will be tempted to believe that healing shame is no different.

In John 9 we encounter shame doing its best to undermine not just the life of one man but of an entire community. The story opens with Jesus coming upon a man blind from birth. His disciples ask, "Who sinned, this man or his parents, that he was born blind?" (v. 2). It is assumed from the beginning that someone is to blame; judgment is the accepted way of life. Shame is evil's ruling scepter. "Neither this man nor his parents sinned," said Jesus, "but this happened so that the works of God might be displayed in him" (v. 3). He counters their question by saying, in part, "It's not about shame. It's about joy!" Already he is turning their attention away from judgment and to possibility. Away from fear to joyful anticipation. But joy has its enemies, and the rest of the story bears this out. Jesus makes mud and applies it to the blind man's eyes, demonstrating that he has no trouble getting close to things that physically evoked shame in everyone; for the man's eyes represented everything about him that was not enough, and everything about the community that only knew how to think of him in categories of fault rather than possibility.

After the man is healed, the trouble begins, the healing having taken place on a Sabbath. First his neighbors are distressed and confused about him. This leads them to bring him before the religious leaders to get their take on things (as if it were the neighbors' job to police such activities). The conversation quickly moves from an inquiry about a healing to an inquisition about the character of Jesus. The Pharisees, unsatisfied as they were with the blind man's assessment (judging, as they did, that his testimony was *not enough*), next call for his parents, who proceed to throw their son under the ecclesial bus, washing their hands of any connection with his story, fearing that they would be put out of the community. The now-seeing blind man is hauled back in to the courtroom, only to call the lawyers out on their hypocrisy. What follows is predictable. "Then they hurled insults at him. . . . And they threw him out" (vv. 28, 34). Shame's mission is complete. The story begins with the judgment of one person—a man born blind—by the disciples and unfolds to reveal how shame has been at work infecting an entire community.

From this we discover at least three things. First, shame is not something that infests only individuals. It is endemic in systems, and any system run by it will seek to maintain its equilibrium. Shame will not share its authority. The blind man's shame is maintained through the organized shame of the community. How is it possible that the only reaction by anyone—the neighbors, the Pharisees or the man's parents—was not immediate, unrestrained joy? This story reminds us that shame is entrenched in our culture. Although individuals may experience healing from shame, as did our formerly blind friend, freedom from it will not be easily maintained apart from being part of communities that support such healing and remind us of the real story we live in, rather than the one shame attempts to narrate.

Natalie endured a horrific rape two years before she first saw me and had not sought professional help prior to our visit. Her shame was so great that she had not even told her parents, fearing that they "won't be able to tolerate knowing about it." What she really feared but was unaware of (the story she was really telling) was that their inability to bear with the gravity of her pain indicated that she was too overwhelming for them. She was not who they needed her to be. There was something wrong with her. Given the depth of her shame, she had no intention of informing her parents or anyone else besides me. "You're a psychiatrist.

I figure you can help me, and then I won't need to tell anyone else."

I informed her that in addition to the hard work she would do in psychotherapy, her shame needed the help of a community in order for it to heal. Her brain would need as many voices as she could handle reminding her that she was loved and cared for, and was not "ruined," a word she often used to describe herself. Though it took several months before she was comfortable doing so, she eventually joined a support group for women who had experienced sexual trauma. Over the course of several months, this group became Natalie's "great cloud of witnesses," a group that in embodied ways—speaking, writing, singing, making meals together, taking hikes—helped transform her shame into a powerful story of redemption, wholeness and creativity. Her shame required a community to realize the fullness of its healing.

It is important to note that these communities can emerge in various settings. They do not form solely within religious circles. They exist in schools, in factories, in neighborhoods, at the office of the technology company, in the coal mine, in the departments of psychiatry in leading medical schools, in art associations, in restaurant kitchens. They are not therapy groups but rather are committed to disallowing shame to be in charge of the system. As we become more acquainted with the shame attendant in each of our individual lives, we see that the whole of shame is larger than the sum of its parts, with each group, no matter its makeup of persons, having its own corporate shame attendant. We push back against the inertia of systemic shame through the weight of a body of people who are collectively engaging in trusting confession, reminding each other of the "great cloud of witnesses." Thus, the need for us to be regularly gathering in places where we are "finding" each other, just as Jesus found the blind man after he had been put out of the synagogue (John 9:35). He found him and gave him the reward for his trust—seeing Jesus face to face.

Which leads to a second discovery. Because shame is an embodied affect, we need more than facts in order to undermine it. For instance, we can read "As Scripture says, 'Anyone who believes in him will never be put to shame'" (Romans 10:11), but still have great difficulty incorporating it into our lives. After he was wounded by an IED, Justin was repeatedly triggered not only by old memories of the war but also by the sight of his prosthesis, which initially evoked overwhelming feelings of shame, first feeling like less of a person, followed by thoughts of the same, given his former fit, athletic physicality. Months of work in the rehabilitation center with the goal of running again (which he eventually reached) did as much to address his shame as his effort directed at his inner life and relationship with God. For we must remember, we are dust and breath, and healing shame will necessarily mean we act differently with our bodies. We will move when before we were literally unable to due to our emotional paralysis. We will speak when before we were silent. We will demonstrate physical agency in the real world, as God did in Jesus by telling people to stretch out their hands (Mark 3:5), take up their mats and walk (John 5:11), and to go and wash (John 9:7). Healing shame is never only an inside job.

Third, we assume that whenever shame is dealt with properly, all interested parties will be happy about it. Our story from John 9 reminds us that this is not always the case. Naming and despising shame, while liberating, will also necessarily reveal all who are actively responsible for propagating it. It would not be hard to imagine, for instance, that when Jesus heals the man, creating space for God's works to be revealed in him (v. 3), he necessarily confronts a community that has understood this man's life in terms of *something that was wrong with him.* There was no evidence of people rushing up to Jesus, urgently asking him to come and heal their blind friend. Healing did not bring comfort and joy to the neighbors. Rather, it brought distress. And whenever genuine acts of goodness evoke responses of distress, you can count on shame being at work, accusing those very neighbors, albeit unconsciously, of their complicity.

The trail from our story in John 9 leads eventually to the community's halls of power where the lawyers, more blind than our unnamed man, make explicit the message that the neighbors had implicitly proclaimed: that the light that comes to heal also hurts our eyes too much and we want that flame to be put out. It might seem odd that in our world healing is met with resistance. But we don't really see this until we begin to hunt down our shame attendant in order to put him out of a job. Healing always requires vulnerability and exposure of our sick and wounded parts, parts often kept hidden and away from our awareness—just as the community in John 9 had kept the blind man out of their consciousness. When they anticipate that the exposure of their shame is pending, many respond fearfully, convinced that they cannot tolerate the discomfort that that exposure necessarily will entail. From the family room to the business lunch to the PTA meeting, there is opportunity for shame to be exposed and healed. And in any of these places, that healing may be met with resistance. For this reason we must routinely engage in confessional communities where we can tell our life stories, reminding ourselves of the joy found in the practice of shame-free emotional nakedness.

We have seen how we can address shame in our interpersonal relationships. We now extend and deepen our exploration to the environments in which we first learn to live and move and have our being. Shame is most insidiously embedded in these institutions, mushrooming to become larger than the sum of its existing parts. And it is there our greatest potential lies for healing, redemption and creativity.

# Redeeming Shame in Our Nurturing Communities

Everything seemed perfect. And every Christmas card would have you believing it. Dominic and Joan had been married for twenty years and had three children who were kind, helpful and hardworking in their school studies. It just didn't make sense when their oldest son, Eric, a senior in high school, decided he wanted nothing more to do with church and was not interested in pursuing a college education. There had been to their knowledge no warning signs. There were no drugs involved. No alcohol. No girlfriend and no hooking up. What had gone wrong?

This was a family who followed Jesus, or at least so they thought. Dominic and Joan were flummoxed at their firstborn's sudden right-angle turn. What to do? After a few weeks of meeting with them, it was clear that this family lived with the motto that you don't have to be perfect, you simply have to do your best. As one of my college professors remarked, possibly one of the least helpful things a parent can tell his or her child is "We only expect you to do your best." No one can do his or her best at everything, for no one has that much time or energy. Shame in this family did not show up as abuse or as a result of someone's alcoholism. There was no divorce on the horizon. Rather, the subtle undercurrent of perfectionism had led to this sudden change in events.

"Have you done your homework?" "Did you fill out those forms I asked you about?" "Have you written your thank-you notes?" Common questions in any family, and on their own they are innocuous enough.

But in Dominic and Joan's home, both consciously and unconsciously, the children lived with the expectation of perfection, as each one told me over time. In the kitchen and the family room roamed a certain shame attendant who reminded everyone—and not just the children—that mistakes are perilous. This was not so much spoken with words but rather with sighs and groans when anyone reported something less than pleasant at the dinner table. Joan was oblivious to her actions, but the children were in unison in their description of their mother's frequent behavior of this kind. What was more, their father usually did nothing to counter it, seemingly equally oblivious to the way these conversations played out.

Finally, Eric had had enough. His announcement that he no longer wanted anything to do with church was as much about his desperate maneuver to breathe as it was about God. But as he told me, how in the world could he possibly please a God who wanted him to do his best in everything? Moreover, Eric wanted answers to questions he had had for several years about faith, about the Bible, about suffering—the usual, reasonable questions anyone would be expected to ask if they were serious about following Jesus. But these queries had always been met with the simple response of "Well, have you prayed about it?" There was little room for the possibility of vagaries when it came to faith. That evoked too much anxiety in Eric's mother, and his father, though devout, had not pursued Eric along these lines, leaving him alone with the unconscious notion that there was too much risk in bringing these concerns to the table.

Eric was insightful enough to recognize eventually that his turmoil over faith arose from worrying that he might not be able to acquire enough information to be sure about this whole Christianity thing. We eventually talked about shame and how easily it works its way into how we decide what to do with Jesus. For if relationship with Jesus is as much about being known as it is about knowing, we soon learn that life with God is not about being right but about being loved. Eric had grown up in a family that taught how to be polite, but not how to comfortably ask questions in a place where it was okay not to have all the answers, or where it was okay for your answers to be wrong.

As it turned out, Eric became the lynchpin around which his family's healing began. The first thing I told his parents was that they did not need to worry about him. Surely God was not worried—he was working, doing everything he could on Eric's behalf. With Eric's permission, I shared with Dominic and Joan what seemed to be some of the basis for his crisis of faith and purpose. We discovered more about Dominic's and Joan's stories, especially those parts they feared would be passed on to their own children: their families' histories of raging alcoholism (Dominic) and anxiety and depression (Joan). In their urgency to not make any mistakes themselves, they found that they were inadvertently passing on to their children the notion that mistakes were forbidden.

## JOY AND SHAME IN OUR FIRST FAMILIES

In this book's introduction, I suggested that it is not enough to simply see shame as a bad thing that needs to be eradicated. Rather, with its healing comes the freedom to more fully live like God in every way he intended, not least being what and how we create in every realm of life. As such, what we have considered from Paul's letter to the church in Corinth (1 Corinthians 8:2-3) is a model for life in every domain, not just the church. So much of our attachment patterns are formed in the context of family, where we have our first experiences of joy and shame. One of the most helpful tools we have for forming secure attachment in our children is making sense of our own stories, bringing out of hiding our own shame. We can move our children toward resilience against shame by sharing with them, when appropriate, our own stories and invite them to tell us theirs. This builds a platform of openness and confidence in relationship rather than certainty in always being right.

When we share our own vulnerabilities with our children, we send a powerful message to their brains that they are not alone in their own weaknesses. Shame would like nothing more than for us to believe we should be able to work out our problems on our own, to do our best at everything and limit our mistakes—we must in order to prevent being abandoned. I do not believe in shoddy work or that we somehow should become inappropriately dependent on others. Far from it. But evil does not tempt us most effectively by offering opportunities for blatant wrong-doing. Rather, it does so through our being so committed to doing our best that we fear we won't be enough.

When we invite our children to talk about their uncertainties and to honestly share our own with them, we make possible the integration of their minds, bringing them not to certainty of knowledge but confidence in relationship. We teach them through our own naked vulnerability that when we suffer—even as Eric did in his existential angst—we learn to persevere, which culminates in the development of resilient character, which leads to hope that does not put us to shame.

For Dominic and Joan, not surprisingly, their son Eric's sudden decision evoked great anxiety not only within but also between them. Eric's "going off the rails" activated within Dominic the impulse to force his son to go to church and at least apply to community college. His heavy-handed approach did little to change Eric's mind. This in turn made Joan even more anxious, fearful that Dominic's anger would only drive Eric further away. Eventually, they were able to recognize that they each had unfinished business of their own. Each of their respective shame attendants was reminding them of how they could have done a much better job parenting and leading them to blame the other for the trouble they were in.

But Dominic began to see that some of his controlling behavior with Eric was really about his need to regulate old feelings of shame around his angry, alcoholic father, who had never taken the time to do much with Dominic except denigrate him when in one of his inebriated states. Joan began to see that her anxiety was tied to her profound sense of inadequacy. Her father had left her mother when she was seven, and her awareness of not being enough was deeply imprinted on her mind. For her, Eric's movement away from church and a college education was not just a choice about lifestyle but a decision to move away from her. And Joan felt abandoned in an altogether novel yet familiar way.

For both Joan and Dominic, the spirit of expecting everyone in the family to do his or her best seemed like a reasonable compromise, a midpoint between the raging control of Dominic's family and Joan's family's tendency to do nothing to upset people for fear of their leaving. Neither

Joan nor Dominic had spent much time revealing to each other the shame and sadness embedded within them. Sure, each knew the facts about the other's narrative, but neither comprehended the full gravity of how the hidden shame each carried was now playing itself out in Eric's choice.

When Dominic and Joan began to tell their whole stories to each other, not just the facts of their narratives but feelings, sensations and images, their shame had fewer dark places to hide. As they each conducted a shame inventory and began to concretely disregard those moments where shame lived and replace them with embodied actions, a curious thing began to happen. Over a period of several months, they reported that their anxiety about Eric was measurably reduced. In fact, they had begun to engage him actively about his questions, validating how hard many of them were to answer, but simultaneously making themselves available to him if he wanted their reflections or advice.

And he did. Eric began to talk more with his parents about their own faith journey. It turned out that Dominic had as many questions as had Eric. Dominic had been too fearful to ask them because the uncertainty and fear he felt were too close to what he had felt as a young boy in the middle of one of his father's alcoholic rages. As long as life was certain, it was not fearful. And for him fear was ultimately about shame, the shame of a father's contempt for his son.

Likewise, Joan began to grow out of her anxiety, albeit slowly, as she felt better understood by Dominic. She started to find her voice and put words to what she was feeling and desired, things she had been too timid to do due to her fear of upsetting someone who would then leave. As she and Dominic continued to grow in telling a new common story, Joan was also able to share with Eric about how her experience of God had long been one steeped in shame, albeit subtle and silent. For her, following God had been about not making mistakes. She did not want to disappoint God, for surely if she did, he would leave. She had never had a community with whom she could share these very intimate details of her life.

Joan grew in resilience, which further enabled Eric to ask questions without feeling as if he would overwhelm her and increase her distress. Instead, as she managed her own distress more effectively, Eric was freed to more genuinely examine his faith without worrying that he would lose his parents in the process.

The journey with this family began when Eric was eighteen. He is now twenty-seven, closer to Jesus than ever and about to complete graduate school. But this has not been a pilgrimage without suffering, and not all stories turn out like this one. I still see them from time to time, as shame is never completely out of the game. But this family's willingness to tell the truth about shame has enabled them to flourish. They now tell a different story from the one they had been telling when I first met them. This is a story of how one family fearlessly disregarded shame, doing the hard, persevering work of listening to the voice of God and living into his delight, something that God wants all of us to experience.

## LEARNING ABOUT SHAME IN THE FAMILY OF GOD

The family of God is the crucible in which we learn what real family is about and in which the *what* and *how* of education is ideally imprinted into our souls, transforming both our life in our biological families as well as all that we learn about our world and our place in it. We have seen how a return to emotional vulnerability—the nakedness of Genesis 2— with our spouse and our children constructs powerful opportunities for increased intimacy and growth in resilience. In living intentionally in this joyful story of vulnerable interdependence, we exercise freedom from the burden of pretense and the maintenance of a false self.

This is the model we also apply to the church. How do we directly address the issue of shame *in* the church so that shame can be healed *through* the church? As it turns out, the process of being known in the context of our vulnerability *within* the church becomes one of the most powerful means of evangelism and healing.

This requires great courage. The very notion of intentionally exposing our shame in a place where we are all ostensibly trying not to do shameful things plays into shame's hand. Who wants to join a community with the reputation (deservedly or not) for being judgmental, even as it preaches against such a thing? What if being this vulnerable results in my experiencing more of the same shame I so long to be free of? These fears of having our shame reactivated and reinforced by the acts we hope will lead to its undoing are part of evil's intention to powerfully use shame in the places where it knows that intimacy—vulnerability—with others and with God will surely lead to its demise.

Although the wellspring for this process is embodied in those who hold formal offices of leadership (pastors, elders, deacons, etc.), it is never limited to them and indeed applies to all within the body of believers. To review, shame positions itself in such a way so as to keep borders tightly closed and vulnerability at a minimum. It teaches us not to reveal weakness, fearing that to do so will lead to our being shamed—the very antithesis of what we need for human flourishing. We have in Jesus one who was willing to put his naked vulnerability on full display, opening himself to all that we in evil's employ could throw at him. He was the first to trust us with himself, revealing himself, risking abandonment in the process. Likewise, in 1 Corinthians 12:23 Paul reminds us that "the parts that we think are less honorable we treat with special honor. And the parts that are unpresentable are treated with special modesty." Here he casts a vision for a community of faith in which we carefully and diligently seek out, protect and honor those who are especially vulnerable and of whom we are easily tempted to be ashamed of, in the same way we are tempted to do the same with parts of each of our inner lives. We do this, as Jesus did with Peter in John, not only in order for them to be given the honor of forgiveness, healing and protection, but also the commission to answer the vocational calling within the church that is uniquely theirs. And Brady needed all of this.

As the pastor of a growing congregation, Brady had been the recipient of many of the typical accolades heaped upon a smart, funny and sensitive preacher. It didn't hurt that he worked hard to keep all of this from going to his head. Not surprisingly, with more people joining his flock every month, there was more work to do, and with that came the inevitable critic, Brady's own personal shame attendant. Brady felt the need to be all things to all people, and as such found it difficult to ask for help. As is the case for many pastors, before long he was in the steep dive of burnout. Responding like so many do when they realize this, Brady worked harder. For some reason, going to a psychiatrist seems to signal that something is terribly wrong in life. When Brady came to see me, it meant to him that he was in trouble. It soon was clear that Brady was not the only one who was working hard to keep his shame attendant happy.

"Who in your church sees to it that you are being cared for?" "Well," he responded, "I have my board of elders, and they're pretty good about asking how I'm doing." "And what do you tell them?" I asked. No signs were posted in the church saying, "Brady: Don't Tell Us About Any of Your Weaknesses—We Don't Want to Know," but Brady could feel it. He sensed it. However, he was not aware that he sensed it until I asked him how it was possible that he had traveled down the path of burnout without anyone taking him aside and asking what was going on. Why had none of his elders asked, "Where are you?" and not stopped until receiving the real answer from Brady. And then the truth tearfully came. "I am so afraid they will see me for who I am and tell me I'm not fit to be here anymore."

Anyone involved in formal church ministry knows this story. It has likely been your story in some fashion at some time in your career. This is the story shame wants to tell. It is the story of hiding fragility. The story of showering those who are smart, gifted and charismatic with approbations, and those who are less so with, well, less. The story in which we have conflicts but are too afraid to face the emotions we anticipate will be waiting for us. These emotions have their source in the shame whose attendant tells us that we are not enough and that Jesus is not enough for us to have this conversation. We won't be able to take it. Furthermore, if we ever imagined that Jesus would be present in that conversation, we might think he could take it, but we don't imagine that he's even there. Instead, we imagine that we will be thrown out, just like the blind man in John 9. "Oh, that would never happen," my left brain tells me, trying to bail me out of my fear. But our reticence to have the hard conversations are evidence that our right brain is far more potent in directing our behavior than our logical left brain is.

Just as in Dominic's and Joan's family, unless leadership of an organization is open to curiosity, open to the idea that unless we are known, what we know doesn't matter, and open to seeking where shame hides, exposing the reality of our naked, vulnerable selves, and disregarding the shame that wants us to hide, we will continue to repeat the interaction that took place in Eden, eventually foisting on our pastors, elders, deacons and staff members what Eve and Adam foisted on each other. "And their eyes were opened . . ." Between our ignorance of and unwillingness to expose our shame, we end up with leadership that turns a blind eye to sexual abuse, interactive styles that foster the maintenance of unspoken caste systems (not least being that between men and women) and doctrinal positions that hold that the proclamation of the gospel leads with the story that we are shameful sinners and follows up with the story that God loves us, rather than the other way round.

We often cope with these undercurrent themes in the same way the first couple did. We seek knowledge. We want to "know." And to know in this case is as much about power as it is about knowledge. Power enables us not only to cope with our deep awareness of weak vulnerability, but also eliminates that weakness from our consciousness. Therein lies part of our desire for larger numbers, bigger stages and greater notoriety for our church. But the larger and more complex the system responsible for carrying the gospel, the easier it is for shame to hide. Our willingness to ferret out shame depends in no small way on plain logistics. And the more people I have to manage, the more difficult it will be to maintain the intimacy that is required to keep my shame attendant in the light. This is not to suggest that, related to church, all things large are bad, merely that it takes greater energy to maintain the awareness of where shame is hiding.

For Brady, it meant having an honest conversation first with two elders he trusted implicitly. This led to further conversations with the rest of them and then the staff. Eventually everyone involved in the church leadership was invited to join a small group committed to engaging these issues on a regular basis. Not everyone participated, and this had its own side effects that had to be addressed. However, Brady no longer felt the pressure to singlehandedly make sure that no mistakes took place on his watch at the church.

In the same way that Joan and Dominic created space for creative, constructive interaction in their home, the leadership in Brady's church

did for its parishioners. Eventually, they made the commitment to train
their small groups in the spiritual disciplines that facilitated greater intimacy, deeper relational connection and the trustworthy space to expose
and disregard shame together. The church grew to be as committed to
being known as it was to growing in numbers. And those who occa-
sionally gathered for worship, but were either skeptical about faith or
simply unaware of the story of Jesus, found in this church people who
were no longer afraid of their shame, and therefore no longer afraid of
what new or different people would bring to them.

The work that Brady and his congregation engaged in initially required heavy lifting. Not because of its complexity but because of the
weight of the shame they feared would fall upon them should they be
honest with each other. For indeed, shame hides most effectively in environments where it ostensibly should be absent. We need only to read
the latest story of a pastor who has sexually abused a parish member or
misused funds for his own purposes to have proof of this. These events
do not happen in a vacuum, but over time congregants and leadership
alike have engaged in microscopic movements of hiding, fearful of the
shame that awaits should they vulnerably expose the reality of their lives.

Within three years of my first seeing Brady, it was clear that his church
was telling a different kind of story. Not one that came from a different
Bible or told of a different Jesus. Instead, they saw in Jesus' forgiveness
the simultaneous disregarding of shame and the opportunity for creating
a new story both as a congregation and as individual parishioners. And
this new story, which begins in the Bible, began to make its way into
places we might not expect the gospel to go: playgrounds, stores, factories, offices. Along the way it became a source of both healing and
transformation for ongoing creative work.

## LEARNING AS A DECLARATION OF VULNERABILITY

As we journey into the world, we participate in new experiences and
learn new parts we are to play in our story. Beginning with the day we
are born, a vital element of that journey is the process of learning. We
learn to recognize our mother's voice. We learn that the thing passing

before our face is our hand and that we can manipulate things with it. Eventually, however, our learning becomes more formalized. While we would reasonably assume that our life of ever-growing discovery is a good thing, shame quickly and efficiently embeds itself there. Hence, it is helpful to explore how shame operates in the process of learning.

Though we usually think of learning as the acquisition of knowledge, we also acquire knowledge for the power it grants us. But acquiring knowledge depends on admitting that we do not know many things, that we need help from others in order to learn. Learning, in fact, is a declaration of vulnerability. We think nothing of this as young children; in fact, we are completely unaware of it. As we grow older, however, we become more distressed. We fear in the future we will be found to not know enough, to have not worked hard enough, to have not scored well enough. We will not be enough. To admit in our culture that we do not have our lives neatly packaged and wrapped, that we are a mess, that we need help from someone else is tantamount to blasphemy. To admit that we do not know something, are not good at something or have made a mistake—to be vulnerably known—is not one of our best skill sets.

In revealing ourselves we risk the shame of not being the smartest person or class or school or nation in the world. We do not wear vulnerability easily or well. In chapter one we learned that many of Jordan's students were quite fearful of not making the grade, literally. As learners, we live as vulnerable creatures who need the presence of others in order for our education to foster an entire panoply of new objects of goodness and beauty.

It is challenging to create a culture of vulnerability that encourages curiosity in a world so wrapped in shame. But curiosity is an important starting point. It begins in the home, with parents guiding their children's natural inquisitiveness and interpreting the world for them as they go. Curiosity depends on being relationally safe (which assumes physical safety). And relational safety rests ultimately on the experience of being known. When we sense the safety engendered by being in the presence of someone we can trust, we are launched into new areas of interest. We are not motivated by the belief we will not fail, but by the conviction that when we make mistakes they will not be our ruin. In an environment where we are unafraid, mistakes are not our enemies but our friends.

In other words, among other things, learning is fearlessly discovering what I know not. One way then to facilitate learning is to offer what might be called creation conversations. These dialogues offer space to discuss where people feel vulnerable or weak—the inevitable nakedness that a child, employee or congregant might be feeling.

One such dialogue took place between the faculty members of a school I recently visited in the Northeast. The teachers were committed to the school's philosophy of making meaningful education available to the economically limited neighborhood where it was located. But the teachers worried that without the support of enough stable families (and the structural support they provide for their children's education), they would not have enough time or energy to meet what felt like over-whelming needs.

As I invited them to talk openly about this, it became evident that many privately harbored the fear of failure. At the same time they believed that everyone else was performing "above grade level." Concealment of their shame led to greater, albeit inefficient, exertion trying to manage all that emotion in addition to doing their work. This creation conversation opened the door for several to have more transparent connection with their principal and peers. Not only were they relieved of their worry, but they could now draw on the emotional and idea resources that a more connected, integrated community can provide.

I call these "creation conversations" because the exposure of the things we are tempted to be ashamed of can lead to creative possibilities. The faculty and staff's achievements would have been inconceivable had they been unwilling to be openly vulnerable.

Of course, this cannot be done cavalierly; there must be careful consideration about the way shame will be flushed out and disregarded. Furthermore, these conversations must be led by persons unafraid of wading into the distressing emotional states of others. But like anything else in life, practice makes permanent, including one's capacity for tolerating those emotional states.

## CHOOSING OUR WORDS OF PRAISE WISELY

The work of Carol Dweck and her collaborators at Stanford sheds light on another approach to how learning best occurs. Briefly, Dweck's thesis is that in education, and in many other realms as well, praise is offered routinely to those who perform well. It is not intuitive that this response on the part of teachers (or coaches or parents or CEOs) could be counterproductive to genuine maturation and creative initiative over the long haul.

What Dweck discovered is that an important predictor of long-term learning effectiveness is the praise of *effort* rather than *outcomes*.[1] In other words, it will do a student (or a child at home or an athlete or my patient or a factory worker) more good when he or she hears something to the effect of "What you are doing is really difficult. I am pleased with how hard you are working at this." Or "You did well—you must have put a great deal of effort in to your work." From an IPNB perspective, this approach addresses the mind as it is truly functioning. We know that learning is about apprehending things we do not know or are not skilled at. For most of us that process entails some degree of work, and the more complex the ideas or tasks we have to complete, the more effort is required. When we hear praise only for having been successful, a curious thing begins to happen in our mind. We begin to associate feeling good with success. Of course, the problem is that we will not always be successful—and we know this, or at least common sense allows us to suspect this.

When I am faced with a problem that I cannot immediately solve, I may become more anxious, because my brain realizes I may be at risk for not being enough, for not being successful and for being shamed because I have failed. If, however, each time I attempt to solve a problem or answer a question my teacher recognizes my effort, I begin to anticipate a different future. If my sense of well-being and connection with my teacher is related to her or his praise for my effort (rather than outcome), even when I am facing a problem I cannot easily solve, I tend not to give up because I anticipate that praise is still coming as long as I put in the effort. This does not mean that praise for good work is unnecessary, unhelpful or detrimental. It is right and good to mention these accomplishments. However, intentionally honoring a person's effort connects to the deeply embedded neural circuits that represent the remembered awareness of the hard work involved. We can cheer as much as we want when our team has won the championship. But the moment of victory is but a temporal sliver of the far-less-glamorous work the team did over the course of the season.

This reveals that in order to directly address shame in the process of education, attention must be paid to the student's effort. What is in play here?

For one thing, we are demonstrating *empathy* when we acknowledge that the work someone is doing is challenging and that we appreciate the effort. We are essentially joining with the student, admitting that the work is difficult and that perseverance is needed in order to master the material. The more I support this person's hard effort in this way, the more she or he feels felt and experiences being known. Certainly the work is hard, and for me to validate that means that the student has the experience of feeling me feeling her or his feelings of just how hard this is.

Without lowering the bar of expectations or attempting to make anything easier for anyone, a leader or parent has the ability to reduce anxiety by reducing the fear of failure. In this way, students who are not necessarily top performers eventually excel, largely because of their perseverance, their resilience. They are less anxious and do well because they are not afraid to fail. The part of their brain that would normally fear the exposure of not being enough is being cared for by an instructor who, via empathy, enables the students to freely do their work and turn their attention away from failure and shame. And who does not desire this?

Our education continues long after we have completed our formal schooling. We long to be more resilient parents, spouses, administrative assistants, tour guides and paramedics. And we will be so if we have others who are engaged with us who, while maintaining worthy expectations, validate that what we are doing is hard work. Not hard in the sense that it requires the complex understanding of quantum mechanics, but in terms of the persistent effort required. We see this progression in what Paul wrote in Romans 5:1-5: suffering (this is hard), perseverance (praise for effort), character (developing resilience) and hope (an anticipated good outcome).

## MINDFUL LEARNING TO COMBAT SHAME

Thus far we have explored the importance of close engagement within our biological and spiritual families as a means of being known and how that enhances our capacity for creativity. We have also seen how empathy strengthens our resilience and willingness to persevere in the face of challenging obstacles. In the course of incorporating these principles as educators, we also open the door to what Ellen Langer labels "mindful learning."[2] She describes several features of what it means to learn mindfully and how mindless learning actually stifles true creativity. One idea in particular that speaks to the issue of shame is her suggestion that real learning takes place when the answers to questions are presumed to be possibilities rather than certainties.

When we are engaged in learning processes in which the questions have only one correct answer, curiosity is silenced. Yes, like Eve and Adam, we reduce our distress most expeditiously by having the right answer, saving us from the shame of being wrong. But in so doing we also close ourselves off to joyful discovery and simultaneously reinforce the shaming fear of making a mistake. When what I am expected to know is limited to the dates of the War of the Roses or the names of its combatants, I stop wondering about all the other things from that conflict that might actually have something to do with real life here and now.

This is not to say that facts are unimportant to daily life (e.g., giving erythromycin instead of penicillin to a patient; a steel beam can hold only so much weight). But the learning process must create the necessary space for movement of our attention and openness to novelty. We tend to practice learning as a regurgitation of memorized facts rather than possible ideas. When the questions are directed toward facts alone, I pay attention to the narrow bandwidth of facts, closing myself off to a vast array of other possible questions and answers. Thus I fail to see goodness and beauty in places I do not look because the answer could not possibly be there. There is, *for certain*, only one right answer to the question. And here shame performs some of its most elegant work.

The idea of certainty, that we can be absolutely sure of facts, was not born in modernity or with the Enlightenment, but it is today most closely associated with scientists such as Sir Isaac Newton. With Newton's new discoveries emerged a set of laws that told us how the universe worked. Things were fixed and unchanging. But with the dawn of quantum mechanics and the wonderings of Werner Heisenberg and Albert Einstein came the notion not of certainty but rather of probability. With everything being relative and composed of particles and waveforms, we learned that the world—right down to that table in your kitchen—is in motion at the level of its most basic elements. We can speak of the degree that motion is occurring, and we might predict with some probability where an object might be, how fast we are traveling or what someone else is thinking, but we cannot know for certain.

This makes us very nervous (and might send us to a psychiatrist!). If I don't know the answer to the question with certainty, I could be wrong. (Hence the proverbial question in class, "Is this going to be on the test?") And I do not associate making mistakes with the joy of learning. Shame takes advantage of this by driving us to certainty in order to protect ourselves from our anticipated humiliation at being mistaken. The more I can know on my own (and not reveal my vulnerable ignorance), the less likely I will be shamed in the process, or so I think. But if we are open to the ideas of probability and possibility and movement as being opportunities for new discoveries, we are opening ourselves to ideas that spring right out of the Genesis account of creation. These ideas speak of a God of action, not of stasis. A God who asks open-ended questions such as "Where are you?" not merely questions with one right answer. And this is not good news for shame, if we are willing to consciously identify its presence and take the proper action to disregard it.

So, we catch a glimpse of how in the context of being known, the affirmation of hard work and the encouragement toward curiosity, shame has more difficulty taking up and maintaining residence in the learning environment. But we must be vigilant, for shame acts early and often, and this is no different in the classroom. For instance, when children are the recipients of shame, even in small increments, in the context of learning to read, it can interfere with the entire scope of their future learning.[3] We know how subtly shame operates. It would be hard to imagine a teacher intentionally planning to shame a student, especially before the rest of a class. But as we have seen in other stories throughout this book, it does not take public humiliation for shame to become operational, and shame doesn't mind that it is not getting the credit in the process.

We have seen how shame can take root—planted in our first family, sprouting in the family of faith, then extending into educational contexts, which become the foundation for how we practice life in our vocational callings. We have also seen how to root shame out of those same foundational systems of life. But we take our family (biological, spiritual and educational) with us to work every day. So we now turn to our final chapter, which focuses on our vocational callings, through which God calls us to steward his good creation. There is no more significant place for us to counteract shame than in those venues where we spend most of our waking hours. In these places we are called to be agents for creating goodness and beauty, but these are the very places where shame is more than willing to do its most effective work.

# Renewing Vocational Creativity

Trained at a prestigious graduate business school, Henry had entered the field of finance. He was interested in using his training to assist small businesses, especially in economically underdeveloped communities. He had accepted a position with a firm that, along with its primary service to wealthy clients who had large portfolios, had launched a division dedicated to smaller targets of investment, just what Henry was looking for. His problem was that his supervisor's primary tactic for helping people perform better was to regularly point out where they needed to improve their work. Henry had quarterly reviews that routinely began with his boss listing the areas where he needed to demonstrate progress, without so much as mentioning Henry's strengths or places of effective guidance for clients. There was no yelling or abject humiliation; simply the constant low-grade hum of disapproval.

His supervisor would also send periodic emails to all of his supervisees offering a performance assessment of the team in general terms, but also of those areas where each team member needed to be improving. This created within the division an unspoken wariness between the team members, each silently critiquing his or her performance vis-à-vis the other, certain that eventually someone would be fired for failing to meet the goals of the division. This was not the way to help a system flourish. Henry lived under these conditions for three years. What had begun with an entire reservoir of enthusiasm eventually drained to nary a drip, his confidence undermined and his interest in the field of helping those in need barely awake. If this was how business worked, he needed to do something very different.

There was no indication that Henry's boss would start each day with the intention of creating a culture of judgment, but that is exactly what emerged. Our tendency toward judgment, however, is ancient, and when we feel vulnerable ourselves, as Henry's supervisor appeared to be, it becomes a handy way for us to cope with our own fear of shame. Judgment strengthens shame's grinding attempt at isolation. In order for me to judge someone, I must create enough distance between us in order to analyze him or her. With that judgment the distance grows. And with enough distance comes isolation. Henry found himself isolated with nowhere to turn in his company. His supervisor did not envision the team as that of a body, as a working whole, but rather as a collection of individuals, each needing to meet his or her quota.

●●●

Becoming more aware of the places where shame hides, in order to disregard it, leads to healing and integration. But what has this to do with other vocational domains of life or the creativity we long to demonstrate there? What does this have to do with software engineering or accounting spreadsheets or how much to ask for my artwork? Let me be clear. There is no substitute for knowing the engineering principles in constructing a building. There is no replacement for learning to tie a proper knot when closing off a surgical procedure. Good relationships won't build a proper ship by themselves. That is not the point. At issue is that *knowing*, which represents the necessary information about how things work, is always in service to *being known*, which represents the relationships for which all of that information matters. And shame works to ruin the creative possibilities of every vocational endeavor by tainting the relationships those endeavors rest on.

Here, *vocation* refers to all I do that requires sustained, repeated effort in stewarding the gifts God has given me, gifts that exist in multiple realms of life. Hence, my vocation involves being a husband, a father, a brother and a friend. It also includes my being a homeowner, a neighbor, psychiatrist, an employer, an elder in my church and a sometime cyclist. God not only gives these domains to me as gifts but also joyfully calls me through them to co-create with him a world of goodness and beauty, inviting others to join me along the way. He does this with all of us. It is not always easy to know how to respond to the multiple callings we may hear, but one thing is sure: shame will not allow us to listen without bringing its dissonance to bear in every way it can.

In the multiple realms of vocational expression shame effectively plays its anticreation role. And the antidote lies in the process of vulnerably being known. In the same way of being known from before the foundation of the world, we were destined to create a world of goodness and beauty, following Jesus' lead in doing things that are the bright shadows of his kingdom that is here and not yet. Vocation—work—in this context is to be equated with creativity. This applies to all vocational expressions in life: parenting, sculpture, engineering, farming, architecture, theology, plumbing, teaching, friendship, music composition, performance and so on. And with each act of joyful creation—right down to the diaper we change in the middle of the night—we proclaim the gospel. This can be done more directly when we speak the name of Jesus, but is often told even more powerfully when told obliquely, like all the best novels and movies. They are the best stories because the storyteller has done the hard work of creating nuance and intimation and curiosity. Hence, we tell the story to our children at the dinner table by speaking of what was the best and hardest part of our day. We tell the story to our employees in the staff meeting by seeking their input on the next significant decision we will make with the firm. And we tell the story to the museum patrons with our sculpture that takes their breath away. But with each act of storytelling, shame is waiting to infiltrate, looking for ways to disintegrate any attempt to create goodness and beauty.

When we resist the disintegration customary of the soul of shame, one byproduct is that we establish space for enhanced creativity. For when the mind is more integrated, it is less distressed. We then have more access to energy for creative endeavors, energy that was being used previously to manage and regulate shame's interpersonal, neurobiological networks. In practical terms, the degree that we are able to ferret out shame in whatever vocational institution we occupy, whether parenting or piloting, we will be more effective and more creative in that domain, not least because we are working to reduce our fear of taking risks, fear rooted in our anticipation of making some relationally catastrophic mistake, fear fueled by shame. Yes, these mistakes can be measured in terms of a misuse of information—prescribing the wrong medicine, entering the wrong algorithm sequence, gathering insufficient supplies— and that misuse can happen for any number of reasons. But their consequences are ultimately measured in terms of whether our life will be okay or not, and that largely depends on some relational dynamic.

## A MODEL FOR VOCATIONAL COMMUNITY

Though it is not the only place to look for how we do this work, Paul's letter to the church in Corinth provides helpful insights to how we can apply what we have learned about healing shame in our everyday lives.

In 1 Corinthians 12–13 Paul addresses the notion of how a body of people function in an integrated fashion. Although he was not a neuroscientist, he paints a picture of a flourishing community, one that is differentiated and linked, an integrated community. He writes these words to a group who at the time were not necessarily in the best shape. There was factional infighting between some who thought others didn't belong, the flaunting of an adulterous affair, and the rather brusque, insensitive approach toward sharing the Lord's meal together. The Corinthian church could easily represent any community today that is gathered around a common purpose.

In 1 Corinthians 12:4-11 Paul describes how the body of Christ develops as a gathering of people with different strengths and capacities.

> There are different kinds of gifts, but the same Spirit distributes them. There are different kinds of service, but the same Lord. There are different kinds of working, but in all of them and in everyone it is the same God at work.
>
> Now to each one the manifestation of the Spirit is given for the common good. To one there is given through the Spirit a message

of wisdom, to another a message of knowledge by means of the same Spirit, to another faith by the same Spirit, to another gifts of healing by that one Spirit, to another miraculous powers, to another prophecy, to another distinguishing between spirits, to another speaking in different kinds of tongues, and to still another the interpretation of tongues. All these are the work of one and the same Spirit, and he distributes them to each one, just as he determines.

That each person brings different gifts to a mission is not novel. But shame has a way of translating *different* into the sense of *better* or *worse*. To the degree that shame has a foothold in my heart, I can unconsciously react to *difference* with judgment directed either at the other or at myself.[1] Even when I am consciously aware of and accept the idea that different people have different tasks, those very structures can activate any latent nidus of shame, especially when things go wrong in a community, and for Henry, things were going very wrong.

In 1 Corinthians 12, Paul makes plain that each member of the body contributes to the welfare of the common good, but also that the body as a whole is the representation of what it means to be truly alive.

Just as a body, though one, has many parts, but all its many parts form one body, so it is with Christ. For we were all baptized by one Spirit so as to form one body—whether Jews or Gentiles, slave or free—and we were all given the one Spirit to drink. Even so the body is not made up of one part but of many. (vv. 12-14)

We cannot thrive on our own. In the same way, IPNB suggests that the mind must function as an integrated whole—differentiated functional parts: attention, memory, emotion, attachment—flexibly linked together. We cannot form the soul of our company, church, school or family well if we fail to see them in this light. Shame's mission is to disintegrate all institutions in the same way it intends to disintegrate individuals, and isolation is no small part of its tactical arsenal.

As followers of Jesus, it is imperative that we routinely do things that help us remember not only which story we are part of but that our story is reflected by our being part of a community. There is no "Jesus and me" option. There is only "Jesus and us." But Paul knows a thing or two about shame, and he next addresses it directly in terms of Jesus' body.

> Now if the foot should say, "Because I am not a hand, I do not belong to the body," it would not for that reason stop being part of the body. And if the ear should say, "Because I am not an eye, I do not belong to the body," it would not for that reason stop being part of the body. If the whole body were an eye, where would the sense of hearing be? If the whole body were an ear, where would the sense of smell be? But in fact God has placed the parts in the body, every one of them, just as he wanted them to be. If they were all one part, where would the body be? As it is, there are many parts, but one body. (1 Corinthians 12:15-20)

He begins where shame begins—with our self-condemnation. In the way that a foot or ear tells itself that it is "not enough," so also we listen to our shame attendant who reminds us of our inadequacies. In so doing we erect barriers within our own minds, cutting off certain parts of our self, those parts we judge to be not enough, from other parts we judge to be more adequate. This is representative of shame's penchant to divide and conquer, and it was coursing through Henry's mind on a daily basis. Paul then turns his attention to the natural course that shame takes, judgment of others.

> The eye cannot say to the hand, "I don't need you!" And the head cannot say to the feet, "I don't need you!" On the contrary, those parts of the body that seem to be weaker are indispensable, and the parts that we think are less honorable we treat with special honor. And the parts that are unpresentable are treated with special modesty, while our presentable parts need no special treatment. But God has put the body together, giving greater honor to the parts that lacked it, so that there should be no division in the body, but that its parts should have equal concern for each other. If one part suffers, every part suffers with it; if one part is honored, every part rejoices with it. (1 Corinthians 12:21-26)

"I don't need you!" This is essentially what our brains say every time we offer even the slightest hint of contempt. It is what Eve and Adam said to each other. It is what we hear every time we are critiqued. This does not mean that each instance is devastating, for we are indeed a rather resilient race. But shame is content in our minimizing any *real* damage here, with our assumption that this is just the way life is. Judgment effortlessly emerges in the forms of sensations, images and feelings as well as thoughts, correlated with the associated neural networks that have repeatedly practiced firing in these same patterns. We don't make these judgment comments so others can hear us—we would be too ashamed to do so. But we do expend a great deal of energy regulating these tendencies. Henry hated to admit the subtle pleasure he felt any time his supervisor mentioned someone else's shortcomings. It helped him cope with his shame and fear of being fired.

But beyond our tendency toward judging others, Paul makes an even more extraordinary statement, especially for his time. He suggests that the weaker parts are indispensable, and that the less honorable parts are to be treated with more honor (vv. 22-23). These "weaker" and "less honorable" elements are understood to carry the weight of shame in that culture. They would normally be seen as disposable, contemptible and worthy of abandonment. But quite counterintuitively, as our IPNB models would also reflect, Paul turns the tables on shame, indicating that the body benefits when its fit and vital parts turn their attention to the more vulnerable parts, seeking them out to create space for them to contribute "indispensably" to the overall health of the body. Here, the IPNB perspective is told as a fundamental theme within the biblical narrative. To flourish, a mind or a community must turn its attention to where shame is hiding in order to create space for even greater growth, even in the way Jesus moves from his place in heaven to join us (Philippians 2:5-8). This is no less true in the context of running a hardware store or a multinational corporation than it is in the church. And it was no less true for Henry's company, something his supervisor did not seem to understand.

First Corinthians 12:15-26, along with Henry's story, sheds light on much of what we have been studying over the course of this book. Notice that (here at least) Paul tacitly suggests that the antithesis to the way of love, which he is about to introduce, is the way of shame. As it was in Eden, it is the affective state out of which judgment—and then the sin that follows—emerges. This recapitulation of Genesis 3 reminds us that when there is an outbreak of shame, no matter how subtle or private, it becomes the base from which evil launches its mission of disintegrating minds and systems in God's good creation.

The passage also highlights the notion that shame is always embodied. It is not an abstract "thing" that exists independent of what we experience in our embodied interactions with other humans. This too is why Paul's metaphor of the body of Christ is so important, for it reminds us that to combat shame requires that we take action in embodied ways.

At the conclusion of 1 Corinthians 12, Paul begins to bring his readers into "the most excellent way," the way of love. Notice that as he transitions into chapter 13, he makes plain that love is neither an abstract idea nor an achievable object, something that can be acquired or realized, as if there is a finite quota. It is a *way*, suggesting a path, suggesting movement, hinting at what he will eventually say, that, "love never fails." It does not fail because it always has another move to make, another gesture toward connection. And there is no end to its movement. We never "arrive," but rather are, and even in the new heaven and earth will be traveling, as C. S. Lewis bids us imagine, "further up and further in."[2] Where shame attempts to push us into static inertia, love bids us to *move*.

Paul then lists a number of noble things we might do, but if they are not done lovingly, they mean nothing.

> If I speak in the tongues of men or of angels, but do not have love,
> I am only a resounding gong or a clanging cymbal. If I have the gift
> of prophecy and can fathom all mysteries and all knowledge, and
> if I have a faith that can move mountains, but do not have love, I
> am nothing. If I give all I possess to the poor and give over my body
> to hardship that I may boast, but do not have love, I gain nothing.
> (1 Corinthians 13:1-3)

In this sense, love is less a noun than an adverb (i.e., *lovingly*), a word that describes the action of a verb, action taken at wisdom's pace. And shame is all about stopping movement, shuttering conversation, crushing creative discovery, acting too quickly or too slowly for fear of making mistakes, and avoiding the repair of ruptures that are inevitable with the mobility of intersecting lives. Furthermore, this section applies to all vocations. If I am the best math teacher, but don't do it lovingly; if I develop the best app, but don't do it lovingly; if I oversee the best children's program of any church in my city, but don't do it lovingly; if I pass important legislation in the Senate, but don't do it lovingly; if I make as much money as possible for the shareholders of my company, but don't do it lovingly—I am nothing. I gain nothing. Paul then proceeds to demonstrate what love is, or rather what it does, again representing it in terms of movement, of action.

> Love is patient, love is kind. It does not envy, it does not boast, it is not proud. It does not dishonor others, it is not self-seeking, it is not easily angered, it keeps no record of wrongs. Love does not delight in evil but rejoices with the truth. It always protects, always trusts, always hopes, always perseveres. (1 Corinthians 13:4-7)

All that we do—parenting, pastoring, farming, playing basketball, carpentry, police work, structural engineering—is done in response to love and shame competing for our attention, wrestling for authority over our memory, emotion, sensations and behaviors. These two dominant affective forces of the universe represent the struggle between good and evil. Within each of us, these two affective states—represented by the presence of the Holy Spirit on one side and our shame attendant on the other—are at war over us and the culture we are making. The Spirit echoes the voice of our Father telling us that we are his daughters and sons, whom he loves and in whom he is pleased. Our shame attendant reminds us in large and small ways that every function of our mind, let alone who we are as a whole, is not enough and has been abandoned. This war occurs in every realm of embodied life.

Finally, Paul reminds us that Jesus' story is one of consummation. God intends to move us from immaturity to maturity, from disintegration to integration, from places where shame hides to where it, being brought into the light, can be disregarded. Then our attention will be drawn to *knowing even as we are known.*

> Love never fails. But where there are prophecies, they will cease; where there are tongues, they will be stilled; where there is knowledge, it will pass away. For we know in part and we prophesy in part, but when completeness comes, what is in part disappears. When I was a child, I talked like a child, I thought like a child, I reasoned like a child. When I became a man, I put the ways of childhood behind me. For now we see only a reflection as in a mirror; then we shall see face to face. Now I know in part; then I shall know fully, even as I am fully known.
>
> And now these three remain: faith, hope and love. But the greatest of these is love. (1 Corinthians 13:8-13)

In other words, we will be aware of (know) God, others and ourselves in the same manner as we experience God's awareness of us. There is no hint of shame in his gaze or his voice. Our attention is drawn so irresistibly to him and how he is attending to us that we lose all awareness of the shame that has for so long kept parts of us hiding in the dark. Toward that end we need to pay attention to the things that are the summation of our lives: faith, hope and love. To live faithfully is to trust, to deeply attune to the presence of the Holy Spirit in whom we live and move and have our being. As we live faithfully, we actively imagine that he *joyfully delights* in being in our presence, and that all we do, we do *with* God, mindful that we live in dependence on him and each other.

Hope is generated as our anticipatory neural networks are shaped by multiple experiences of trust being affirmed and rewarded. To the Roman followers of Jesus, Paul writes:

> Therefore, since we have been justified through faith, we have peace with God through our Lord Jesus Christ, through whom we have gained access by faith into this grace in which we now stand. And we boast in the hope of the glory of God. Not only so, but we also glory in our sufferings, because we know that suffering produces

perseverance; perseverance, character; and character, hope. And hope does not put us to shame, because God's love has been poured out into our hearts through the Holy Spirit, who has been given to us. (Romans 5:1-5)

Note the progression from suffering to perseverance to character to hope, and hope of this sort does not put us to shame. In the story the Bible tells, hope is not magic. It does not appear out of thin air on our emotional doorstep. It requires effort to develop. We must do the some-times painfully hard work of perseverance, of looking at shame re-peatedly and disregarding it repeatedly. In so doing the resilience of character—the flexible, adaptive, coherent, energized and stable states of integration—emerges as the byproduct of our transformation, which enables us to remember a different future. This is a hopeful future, God's future, that, as N. T. Wright suggests, has in Jesus already moved forward into our present, renewing everything about it, while pointing to what is coming. And this hope, this imagery of being joyfully known, leaves no room for shame.[3]

Without shame, love, the greatest of all that remains, liberates us not only to behave kindly, patiently and all the rest, but also to create as God intended from the beginning. I mentioned earlier that love and shame are the two fundamental affective states warring for our souls. Of course, this oversimplifies the case. It is not as if shame is the only emotion that gives us trouble, and love houses virtually every emotion that leads to constructive, integrating behavior. The point here, however, is that in many respects life is not that complicated. In any instant it boils down to microdecisions we make that generally move us in one of two direc-tions: a more integrated, resilient life of connection with God and others, or a more disintegrated, separated, chaotic and rigid life. Every minute of every day we choose between shame and love.

But we must not forget that these are not mere artifacts of existence, unless we are living in the common story that our culture tells, the story in which there is no God and in the end everything will go dark. But if we believe we are part of a great tapestry that God is weaving, then every

moment we choose to intentionally live vulnerably, exposing our shame
in the context of safe, healing communities, we, with God's help, place
one more stone in building the kingdom of God, which is both now and
not yet. In the process we tell the great story of hope, trust and joy, despite the hard work that is necessary to bring a great drama to its climax.

## Renewing Our Vocational Mind

We can learn much from the brain and the notion of integration that can
be applied to the myriad vocational domains, intentionally telling the
story of God in ways that are naked and unashamed. In the same way
that the prefrontal cortex (PFC) is necessary to attune to multiple functions of the mind, and thereby leading to a state of integration, so also
every system needs leaders committed to the differentiation and linkage
of the functional parts of that system. The neurons that correlate with
our attentional mechanism reside in the PFC. These connect various
functional neural networks to each other (i.e., memory, emotion, our
ongoing narrative, our ever-changing states and our awareness of other
minds we interact with). In this way the PFC functions much like the
mind's leader. In this region of the brain, to the extent it is possible, what
we sense, image, feel and think are brought to conscious awareness—especially those features we may find undesirable, such as unpleasant emotions—in order to make sense of them and connect them with other
parts of the mind. In this way each emotion, sensation, feeling and
physical action are given their proper place and meaning, contributing
to the overall health of the mind. Leadership, then, within the activity of
the mind, could be considered to be that function of the PFC which, *with
intention*, makes possible for each element of the mind to do what it was
created to do as a differentiated, linked part of a larger whole. And this
opens the door to creativity beyond our imagination.

This then provides a template for what leadership does in human
systems, in the vocational realms we occupy. Leadership can be understood as enabling, *with intention*, those who are relationally close, and for
whom the leader has responsibility, to flourish—to joyfully do the good
works God has foreordained. According to Dave Schrader, leadership is

not limited to, nor does it automatically emerge out of, hierarchical organization. Therefore, everyone is a potential leader.[4] Any system that takes this approach to leadership will require intention and perseverance, and will bear the fruit of creating goodness and beauty.

Shame is aware of what this kind of leadership can do, and will give it no quarter. It is well aware that leadership is enhanced when we are willing to live more in line with our created state of vulnerability by revealing the truth of who we are. And eventually that truth will include those areas in which we don't have the answers or when we need help. This is especially true when we are in relatively higher positions, a situation in which Gavin found himself.

"I just don't see that happening." I had been consulting with Gavin about his business. We had explored his concerns about his company and particularly about his managers who were complaining about their workload over the last quarter. Gavin was conscientious and a hard worker. He cared about his employees and had always strived to provide the support they needed to carry out their assigned projects.

But something had changed in the last six months. With the acquisition of the company's first large government contract, there was more at stake. More money. More pressure to perform. More risk for failure and by extension for what Gavin anticipated would be some form of public corporate humiliation. It was clear that he was overwhelmed. It was also clear that to admit that would require great courage on his part. He perceived himself to be a self-starter and felt personal responsibility to find solutions for problems that came his way, even for those that at times belonged to others. Whenever he, the unstoppable force, encountered the proverbial immovable object, the object always moved. But for some reason, this one wasn't budging.

As part of our consultation, I invited Gavin to tell me his story. The nature of the answer to such an open question itself can be revealing. "What do you mean, 'Tell me your story'? What part of my story do you want to know?" As we have been learning, we are telling stories all the time, but we often don't have that much practice telling them to people who genuinely want to know much about us beyond our vital statistics or our latest brilliant plan for saving the company. At first Gavin somewhat clumsily patched together his version of what he thought I wanted to hear. Not surprisingly, his story included a great many successes, about which he was humble. He was married, with two children. He was a devout follower of Jesus and was involved in a local community of fellow believers. He was in relatively good health. He had, to his knowledge, few large problems looming on the horizon, apart from what brought us together. Along with that, though, it was clear he did not easily reveal weaknesses.

I inquired about what experiences he had asking for help as he grew up. "Well, people could ask for help. I helped people all the time, and my parents helped me." Gavin was the oldest of five siblings, and he took his role as firstborn seriously. He cared deeply for his siblings, and this took on particular significance after his father died unexpectedly when Gavin was sixteen. It was not immediately evident to him that asking for help was to him experientially separate from helping someone. For in the wake of his father's death, Gavin found himself feeling responsible in heightened ways, especially given his mother's sadness, which lasted several months.

"What do you think about weakness?" I asked. Gavin was bright and insightful, and he offered a response that was reasonable. "Everyone has weaknesses. It's good to know what they are so you can work on them to strengthen them." I asked how he approached weakness in his company. "We do everything we can to support people, to give them the development and training opportunities they need to be better at what they do." "And what about you?" I asked. "Who is responsible to help you with your weaknesses?" He thought for only a moment. "Well, I am, of course. Who else's job would it be? I mean, I own the company."

Gavin's is a common story with a common theme. The longer we talked, the more clear it became that, although his life was flourishing on many levels—despite his having been left fatherless at an early age—he was hovering over a yawning abyss that would soon swallow him unless he changed the way he was approaching not only his business but his life.

## EXPOSED TO BE HEALED

Elsewhere we have considered the notion that one of shame's most acute byproducts is the fear of exposure, the very thing that, paradoxically, is required for shame's healing. It requires great courage to reveal ourselves in the face of the abject terror that we will be seen and then rejected. To expose our real self—our weaknesses, flaws, mistakes and brokenness, along with our desires, needs, and hopes—to others who may hurt us involves the risk that we may be criticized, judged and dismissed.

I wondered aloud what Gavin thought of telling his managers that he felt overwhelmed and needed not only for them to work more efficiently—he needed their ideas. He was, in fact, *needy*. The very word was off-putting to him, conjuring images seeming to others to be pathetic. To this suggestion he responded with his comment "I just don't see that happening." He was sure that once they knew he did not have all the answers, they would no longer respect him as a leader. It was foreign to him that one of the most empowering things he could do for his own health, the health of his managers and for the company was to come clean about feeling "in over his head." We explored what emotion was evoked within him in his current situation. With reflection, he listed the following: fear, alone, stupid, powerless. Pausing to move more deeply into what those feelings represented, I wondered what he imagined he would feel after telling his employees the truth. "I know this might sound silly, but I would feel so ashamed."

Once again shame was the undercurrent preventing Gavin from telling his whole story and potentially finding liberation for his company in the process. And so we spoke about the nature of shame and what it would be like for him to confront it directly by sharing his full story with his managers. Although he could see the logic in it, Gavin was suspicious of such a tactic. The longer we talked, the more he came to see that in both his business and in other areas of his life, although he liked to think of himself as confident, secure and competent, he was now feeling vulnerable. And the vulnerability he sensed at his work was beginning to seep into other areas of his life.

This is how shame works, viral in nature as it is. It creates a deep fear of vulnerability. When our response is to retreat and hide, working harder to demonstrate our impenetrability, shame spreads to other regions. Not unlike what happens if an abscess is not lanced, the infection spreads to other tissue through the most undefended path. Gavin admitted that since he was spending so much more time trying to figure out how to solve his company's problems, he was more irritable at home with his wife and children, he spent less time playing poker with friends, and his typical rhythm of exercise and spiritual practices had been out of sync. He was not interested in vulnerability. He was interested in solutions. He wanted a more fail-safe maneuver to relieve him of how vulnerable he felt.

Essentially, Gavin was telling himself that he was not enough, that he did not have what it took to reveal his limits. Gavin's shame attendant was working full time and not giving an inch. Several weeks after our meeting, when he was running out of ideas and patience, not least with himself, Gavin took the courageous step of inviting his most senior managers into his world of neediness and embarrassment. He was shocked at what he found.

His managers, to a person, responded with relief and energy, with no condemnation whatsoever. They had wanted to be included far sooner in the process of figuring out the solution to the company's troubles. They did not speak of their disappointment in him for not having all the answers (something he dreaded), but rather of how impressed they were that he was willing to risk admitting his shortcomings. It took several weeks, but eventually between his managers and some other trusted colleagues he also revealed his problems to, the company was able to find its legs and once more become productive. Going forward Gavin found new ways to effectively create a product his client was pleased with, enhance the morale in his company, and feel less overwhelmed with the weight of it all by seeking shame where it was hiding in his business soul and disregarding it, and by joining a community where he no longer felt alone. This reduced his and everyone else's anxiety, and enabled them to consider creative means to once again allow the company to flourish.

Gavin's story reminds us that God is at work in our work. Jesus is bringing redemption and healing through vocation. And shame has every intention of disintegrating that endeavor. Where we are willing to do the work of attuning to its presence in order to scorn it, and to bring those parts of our minds and vocations into the light for care, discipline, and encouragement through the joyful, just, and merciful role of leadership, we will find ourselves amazed at what unfolds. Those we shepherd, for example, will flourish in a culture that exposes shame, allowing room for healing and creativity.

It does not matter what vocation we are called to. If we have any unfinished business with shame, it will seek us out, all the while attempting to remain hidden as it does so. It will find us in our mistakes, our unrepaired relationships and our drivenness to control our emotional states in isolation rather than through the interpersonal regulation we find in community. Our shame attendant wants us to think, feel, sense and image that we are not enough, just as Gavin's had, and just as evil did with Adam and Eve so long ago. It will tempt us to tell a story in which we are on the brink of abandonment and must do everything we can—on our own—to prevent that from happening. It will seek to divide and conquer our sensations, images, feelings, thoughts and behaviors from one another, leaving us in a disintegrated heap. It will reinforce itself by allowing us to feel ashamed for feeling shame in the first place. It will convince us that to trust others with our most precious feelings will be our emotional death.

This is the business of shame. Its mission is to thwart all intentions to create a world of goodness and beauty, especially through our vocational callings. After reading this book, it would be tempting to think that shame is the only thing we need pay attention to, and if we do, life will flourish. Shame is certainly not the only evidence of broken relationships. But precious little evidence suggests that shame is not the root cause of much that we experience of the kingdom of darkness.

The gospel tells a very different story: We are God's sons and daughters in whom he is very pleased. He is delighted to be in our presence. And it is love's business to draw us together as a people in an integrated whole of differentiated, linked parts who are capable of amazing creativity. No one is left behind or left out. But we are not blind to the fact that we have different work to do, with some being more visible than others.

How would it look to live as an integrated people in real life? How would the renewing of our minds (Romans 12:1-2) alter what happens in my family? How does the literal rewiring of my brain, the embodied alteration of my neural networks and my physical behavior, strengthen and make more permanent the witness of a church in its community? What would be the outcome of explicitly addressing shame in educational contexts? For indeed, teaching and learning begins at home, is made manifest in the family of faith, is formalized in our educational institutions, and hopefully never ends. Given that it occupies virtually all of life, it would be irresponsible for us to ignore how shame plays a particularly destructive role in these institutions.

## WHAT STORY WILL OUR SOUL TELL?

We have now come full circle. We have explored the fundamental nature of shame and have seen that it is no mere artifact but rather an intentionally wielded element of the human experience that evil uses to silently and subtly disintegrate our minds, relationships and communities. We have also seen that healing shame requires our willingness to seek it out (following Jesus' example) rather than waiting for it to find us in our naiveté. Finally, we have seen how our storytelling practices begin at home, are honed in the family of God and are then taken with us into every vocational realm we occupy. In this way we see how evil's intention for shame is not simply to make our interpersonal lives miserable; it wants to destroy everything about the world that God intended for goodness and beauty. It wants to cripple our creativity as artists and engineers and teachers as much as it wants us to merely feel bad about ourselves.

This book is about shame. About its soul—and its attempt to dismantle ours. But mostly this book is about telling a new story, a story of hope and creativity, one that scorns shame in order to imagine new minds, new possibilities and new narratives, all of which point to the new heaven and earth that we believe Jesus is surely bringing. We have seen that healing shame through God's coming in Jesus is not only something that regenerates our relationships between ourselves and God, family, friends and enemies, but so much more. It is one of the most important features in liberating us to tell a new story rather than the one shame has been trying to tell from the beginning. It infuses us with the courage to imagine new ways to create in our respective vocations, just as God dreamed of when he first considered making us, when he first envisioned us living like he lives.

This healing and renewed potential for creativity can only be accomplished in deeply connected community. We cannot do this alone. The prospect of forming or finding that type of community can seem daunting. Where am I going to find those who will help me tell my story, who are willing to do the things we have explored in this book? These are reasonable and sometimes hard questions. It is easy to become discouraged when the possibilities described in these pages seem unlikely to be realized. I should know. For truly, there are times when, despite having a network of relationships who are willing to do this hard work with me, I still hear shame knocking on the door of my heart more loudly than I would like.

But shame does not get the final word in the story Jesus is telling—the one he invites us to participate in as coauthors, the one in which God's delight commands our attention far more than does our shame. Moreover, I want to encourage you, despite your fear, to enter into this life of telling a different story than the one shame wants you to believe. I do so because I know from my own experience that it is worth it. Despite how hard the work can sometimes feel, it is worth it. Its worth it to know the liberation of retelling my story so very differently from the way shame would have it be told. I do not want to be alone on this journey, and so I ask you to join me. I look forward to how, together, God will enable us to retell our stories as part of the great Story he longs for all of us to join.

# Acknowledgments

When it comes to acknowledging people for their help and contribution to a writing project, the lines are fuzzy. For indeed, there have been what seems like an infinite array of interactions with who knows how many people who have supported and informed the work of bringing this book to life. People who are living, pulsating testimonies to the notion that yes, shame is real, but also to the even greater notion that because of God's yes in Jesus, shame does not need to have the talking stick when we tell the stories of our lives.

And so I begin with the many who have opened their lives to me and granted me the deep honor of being present with them in the center of their stories—even places of significant shame—to realize the joy and liberation that comes through being known. That list starts with my patients, who are anything but nameless and faceless, and who daily help me believe in a God who has cleared his throat and is telling a story of beauty and goodness in the face of evil's attempt to do otherwise. In addition, over the last several years as I have been invited to speak in so many different places, I have been the recipient of the unfathomable gift of new relationships. These people have honored me by inviting me into their communities, allowing me to be part of their journey as they do the hard work of scorning shame, turning to new avenues of vocational creativity, and providing deep comfort and encouragement to me on the path to completing this book. Those communities include but are not limited to Corinth Reformed Church in Hickory, North Carolina; the gathering at the Friends Pastors' Sabbath Retreat at Horn Creek, Colorado; the good people at Burke Consortium; Barnabas International; the Office of the CIO, US Department of the Navy; Kent Annan and Haiti Partners; David Jenkins and his colleagues at the Center for Counseling and Family Studies at Liberty University; Trinity Forum Academy; Bill Haley and Corhaven; Michael and Amy Monroe and Tapestry; Michael Gulker and the Colossian Forum; Steve and Gwen Smith and Potter's Inn; and so many more. Indeed, if I have not mentioned you, it is only because I can't list everyone. But if I have been with you, know that you are one of the important reasons this book is in your hands.

One community deserves special mention, however. Over the past three years I have been privileged to serve with a team of gifted friends who are creating their own pocket of goodness and beauty in the world called Seasons Weekend. No group has more effectively held, shaped and transformed me in the time of writing this book than this, my freshly acquired family of intimacy. Thanks, then, to Nicole Johnson and her vision for bringing together a company of fellow pilgrims whose very breath has so crucially helped bring forth the text on these pages.

While on a speaking engagement in New Zealand, my new friend Scott Milne looked at me as we were debriefing our time there and said, "Everyone has one book. You have done that. You need to write the next book. The book on shame must be done." I seem to respond well to marching orders that are expressed as strong, confident encouragement. That's what I received that day on the North Island. I am so, so grateful for Scottie and Jennie and their infusion of kindness, joy, and hope during our stay in New Zealand.

Once again, my agent Leslie Nunn Reed has done it. She has continued to be a calm, guiding presence as I navigate the ever-changing world of publishing. I can't imagine there being a book I would ever write in which at the end I am not thanking her for all she does.

For all the people at InterVarsity Press who have made this project possible I am so very grateful. For Dave Zimmerman, who while at IVP was the first to take on and introduce the concept. For Jeff Crosby, whose unmitigated enthusiasm, joy and (in his words) bullishness about the project gave me more confidence than he might know. There is absolutely nothing like being wanted. (Well, not like Jesse James was wanted, but you know what I mean.) Thanks to Al Hsu who has provided needed support, especially in a time of editorial transition.

And then there is Helen Lee. What an absolute delight to have an editor so capable of effectively guiding the process with directness, kindness and humor—while tolerating my neuroses about writing all at the same time. To whatever degree the writing found herein has been at all good, it stands that it is to no small degree due to Helen's work. I look forward to any chance I have to work with her in the future.

Finally, it is fair to say that the voices of many of my closest family, friends and colleagues are never far away from me. They have been great encouragements to me as well as much of the inspiration for writing as they have spoken on many occasions of their anticipation of the release of this book. Thank you to so many who have provided the energy when I most needed it to do my part to make this work a possibility. My life is only what it is because you are in it.

# Discussion Guide

## CHAPTER 1: OUR PROBLEM WITH SHAME

1. What features of shame (emotional nature, judgment/condemning in tone, hiding, self-reinforcing, isolation/disconnection) feel familiar to you?

2. Can you name some examples of experiences in which you have encountered one or more of those features?

3. What is your immediate response to considering answering question 2?

4. What is your impression of the counterintuitive actions necessary for shame's healing?

## CHAPTER 2: HOW SHAME TARGETS THE MIND

1. Describe your reaction to the working definition of the mind. What parts of it seem novel? What parts are helpful?

2. Which of the nine domains of integration of the mind seem to generate curiosity within you? Which seem to generate discomfort?

3. In what parts of your mind and life do you long to know greater *integration* as this chapter has described it?

4. How well do you pay attention to what you pay attention to? What challenges does this pose for you?

5. What memories, either implicit or explicit, do you find reflect the experience of shame?

6. In reading this book, what role have you discovered that emotion plays in your life?

7. What do you suspect is the form of attachment you experience with your closest friends? How does it strike you that "your" story is best understood in terms of how it is shared with others?

## CHAPTER 3: JOY, SHAME AND THE BRAIN

1. What is your experience of joy in your daily life? What would it be like to keep a record of the small moments in your day in which joy is present but out of your awareness?

2. Who are the people who propagate joy in your life by consistently demonstrating their delight upon encountering you?

3. Describe a time when your experience of shame disintegrated your sense of joy and curiosity. What were the physical, emotional and cognitive consequences that you can recall?

4. What features of shame that you have encountered in this chapter do you find familiar?

5. Considering the notion of the mind's domains of integration in chapter two, which domains seem most likely to become "disintegrated" for you upon encountering shame? What is the evidence for this in your experience?

## CHAPTER 4: THE STORY OF SHAME YOU ARE LIVING

1. How did it strike you to discover that you are telling your story at all times?

2. The book indicates that we tell stories with more than just words. What elements of storytelling (sensations, images, feelings, thoughts, words, actions) do you find yourself paying attention to—and necessarily responding to as well?

3. What part of your story were you surprised to find that you are telling—all the time, with sensations, images, feelings or thoughts?

4. Which form of your story (large, medium, small) do you find yourself paying the most attention to?

5. What part of your story that was told before and early after you were born seems to have a significant influence over how you think about your life now?

6. In what story do you believe you are living? What would the evidence of what courses through your mind regularly reveal about the large, medium and small story in which you believe you are *really* living?

7. Who are the people who regularly enable you to tell your story well by listening just as well? If you do not have relationships such as these, who currently is in your life with whom you would like to form that kind of relationship?

8. Whose story do you help to tell by being a good listener?

9. Describe your shame attendant. What does she say to you? How does he look at you? His tone of voice? Her frequency of judgment?

10. In what ways does your shame attendant "shear off" your experiences of joy and creativity?

## CHAPTER 5: SHAME AND THE BIBLICAL NARRATIVE

1. What do you *feel* when you consider that "the man and the woman were naked and they felt no shame"?

2. Imagine the unfolding nature of the serpent's conversation with the woman. What do you imagine she would be feeling as she progressed through that encounter?

3. How does the notion that shame entered the story in the Garden of Eden before the couple ate from the tree of the knowledge of good and evil strike you?

4. In what way does the propagation of shame in Genesis 3 feel familiar to your own life?

5. What tactics do you employ to hide? From whom do you hide? With whom—on your best days—do you wish you could be fully transparent?

6. Who are the people who come calling to you, inquiring of your whereabouts, as God did with Adam?

## CHAPTER 6: SHAME'S REMEDY: VULNERABILITY

1. What has been your experience of making yourself intentionally vulnerable?

2. What are some behaviors you employ to avoid being vulnerable?

3. What images come to mind and what emotions do you feel when you consider that God has come to find us? To be known by us? To remain with us?

4. In what ways does shame "silently and subtly" make its way into your life?

5. What parts of your life do you fear vulnerably exposing to another?

6. Consider choosing two to three people to whom you would vulnerably expose those parts of your life for which you feel shame. Who would they be?

7. List one to three stories/events of your life that you would share vulnerably with those people.

## CHAPTER 7: OUR HEALING CLOUD OF WITNESSES

1. Who would be those, living or deceased, who make up your own "great cloud of witnesses"?

2. What difficulties do you foresee in forming your own cloud of witnesses in which you can effectively scorn shame?

3. What sensations, images, feelings, thoughts or behaviors pose as the more prominent distractions that draw your attention away from a joyful, welcoming, inviting triune God and toward shame?

4. What acts of imagination will you begin to practice as a means of shifting your attention away from shame and toward Jesus?

5. Practice taking the shame inventory. Note what you are tempted to feel and do whenever you make a mark on your card. What do you sense

and feel when you merely shift your attention away from the shaming event with its accompanying condemnation and back to your life?

6. What do you begin to notice as you persevere, upon encountering an accusing moment of shame, in turning your attention instead to the images and sounds of "You are my beloved son/daughter; I am so pleased that you are on the earth and that I have the privilege of being your Father"?

7. To whom are you able to confess the events of your life so as to hear, when necessary, "You're right. You're wrong"?

8. Name the different communities you occupy (family, work, friends, faith fellowship, sports, etc.). What is the general posture of each of these groups in regard to vulnerability? To revealing hidden shame?

9. Communities of healing are not limited to the church. In what place(s) do you have a community that serves as a place of healing?

## CHAPTER 8: REDEEMING SHAME IN OUR NURTURING COMMUNITIES

1. What memory do you have of joy in your early developmental life?

2. Where have you experienced shaming experiences in your family of origin?

3. In what ways did the family in which you were reared offer healthy ways of addressing shame?

4. How much did your family practice talking about feelings, especially those associated with feeling vulnerable?

5. Where do you experience joy being emphasized in your current encounter within the church setting? How often do you consider joy to be a significant element of the story of the Bible?

6. What experiences have you had in the church in which shame played a significant role?

7. Where have you witnessed shame being "scorned" and healed within the community of faith? What concrete steps were taken to enable this to happen?

8. What ways do you recall shame beginning to emerge in your memory of your educational experience?

9. Can you remember a teacher, coach or professor who was an effective educator without using shame as a tool of the trade? If so, what specific thing(s) did she or he do that were helpful?

10. Describe your impression of Dweck's notion that it is relatively more helpful to place emphasis on praising effort than on praising outcomes.

11. Describe your response to Langer's concept that effective learning is more about possibilities than certainties.

12. Where do you currently find the pursuit of learning something new being held back by shame?

## CHAPTER 9: RENEWING VOCATIONAL CREATIVITY

1. What are the domains that make up the collection of your vocational callings?

2. What are the vocational domains, or parts of domains, in which you desire to be more willing to take risks, to risk making mistakes, to be creative?

3. How does your shame attendant interfere with God's calling for you to enter into creative stewardship?

4. Who in your life has fostered an environment that has enabled you to become a more effective leader? What have been the explicit, concrete actions that person has taken to facilitate your growth?

5. In your place of work (where you spend the most hours of your day or week), to what degree does the general culture reflect one of shame? Of invitation to vulnerability and creativity? What explicit behaviors embody any of these features?

6. After reading this book, and chapter nine in particular, about which realms of vocational creativity are you finding yourself to be more curious? Upon noticing such curiosity, what is your immediate embodied response?

7. What concrete steps are you willing to take to realize greater exploration of the vocational areas about which you are becoming more curious? What are the sensations, images, feelings and thoughts that enter into your awareness that represent shame's attempt to stop such curiosity?

8. What community can you begin to build that will support the story of new creation that you, in answering God's call to join him, are beginning to tell?

# Notes

**CHAPTER 1: OUR PROBLEM WITH SHAME**

[1]Daniel J. Siegel, *The Developing Mind* (New York: Guilford, 1999), pp. 117-20.

**CHAPTER 2: HOW SHAME TARGETS THE MIND**

[1]Curt Thompson, *Anatomy of the Soul* (Carol Stream, IL: Tyndale House, 2010), p. 5.
[2]See the March, July, October and December 2012 issues of *Scientific American*.
[3]Daniel J. Siegel, *The Mindful Brain* (New York: W. W. Norton, 2007), pp. 4-5.
[4]Alex Eccleston et al., "Epigenetics," *Nature Insight* 447, no. 7143 (2007): 396-440.
[5]Daniel J. Siegel, *Mindsight* (New York: Bantam, 2010), pp. 71-75.
[6]Diana Fosha, Daniel J. Siegel and Marion F. Solomon, *The Healing Power of Emotion* (New York: W. W. Norton, 2009), pp. vii-xiii.
[7]Louis Cozolino, *The Neuroscience of Human Relationships* (New York: W. W. Norton, 2006), pp. 86-87.
[8]Siegel, *The Developing Mind*, pp. 77-88.
[9]Timothy Wilson, *Strangers to Ourselves* (Cambridge, MA: Harvard University Press, 2002), p. 6.

**CHAPTER 3: JOY, SHAME AND THE BRAIN**

[1]Leo Tolstoy, quoted in Peter Sekirin, *Divine and Human* (Grand Rapids: Zondervan, 2000), p. 18.
[2]C. S. Lewis, *The Weight of Glory and Other Addresses* (New York: HarperCollins, 1949), pp. 35-38.
[3]Allan Schore, *Affect Regulation and the Repair of the Self* (New York: W. W. Norton, 2003), pp. 37-41.
[4]E. James Wilder, Edward Khouri, Chris Coursey and Sheila D. Sutton, *Joy Starts Here* (East Peoria, IL: Shepherd's House, 2013), pp. 6-8.
[5]Carol Dweck, *Mindset: The Psychology of Success* (New York: Ballantine, 2006), pp. 70-74.
[6]Robert Browning, *Selected Poems*, ed. Daniel Karlin (New York: Penguin Classics, 2000), p. 115.

[7]Michael Lewis, *Shame: The Exposed Self* (New York: Simon & Schuster, 1992), pp. 91-94.

[8]Ibid., pp. 94-96.

[9]Schore, *Affect Regulation*, pp. 154-63.

[10]Daniel J. Siegel and Mary Hartzell, *Parenting from the Inside Out* (New York: Penguin, 2003), p. 215.

[11]Silvan Tomkins, *Affect Imagery Consciousness: The Complete Edition* (New York: Springer, 2008), pp. xviii-xix.

[12]John Gottman, *The Seven Principles for Making Marriage Work* (New York: Three Rivers Press, 1999), pp. 29-31.

[13]Daniel J. Siegel, *The Developing Mind* (New York: Guilford, 1999), p. 279.

## CHAPTER 5: SHAME AND THE BIBLICAL NARRATIVE

[1]Lesslie Newbigin, *The Gospel in a Pluralist Society* (Grand Rapids: Eerdmans, 1989), pp. 8-11.

[2]Curt Thompson, *Anatomy of the Soul* (Carol Stream, IL: Tyndale House, 2010), pp. 207-20.

[3]C. S. Lewis, *A Grief Observed* (New York: Bantam Books, 1976), p. 9.

[4]Michael Polanyi, *Personal Knowledge* (Chicago: University of Chicago Press, 1958), pp. 272-75.

[5]David Benner, *The Gift of Being Yourself* (Downers Grove, IL: InterVarsity Press, 2004), p. 20.

## CHAPTER 6: SHAME'S REMEDY: VULNERABILITY

[1]Brené Brown, *Daring Greatly* (New York: Gotham, 2012), pp. 32-56.

[2]Ibid., pp. 111-71.

[3]Daniel J. Siegel, *The Neurobiology of We: How Relationships, the Mind, and the Brain Interact to Shape Who We Are* (Louisville, CO: Sounds True Audio Learning Course, 2008).

[4]Curt Thompson, *Anatomy of the Soul* (Carol Stream, IL: Tyndale House, 2010), pp. 16-18.

[5]David Benner, *The Gift of Being Yourself* (Downers Grove, IL: InterVarsity Press, 2004), pp. 61-70.

## CHAPTER 7: OUR HEALING CLOUD OF WITNESSES

[1]I explore the IPNB features of this text in Curt Thompson, *Anatomy of the Soul* (Carol Stream, IL: Tyndale House, 2010), pp. 226-28.

## CHAPTER 8: REDEEMING SHAME IN OUR NURTURING COMMUNITIES

[1]Carol Dwek, *Mindset: The Psychology of Success* (New York: Ballantine, 2006), pp. 70-74.

[2]Ellen Langer, *The Power of Mindful Learning* (New York: Perseus, 1997), pp. 133-35.

[3]Donald L. Nathanson, interview by David Boulton, *Children of the Code*, September 8, 2003, www.childrenofthecode.org/interviews/nathanson.htm.

## CHAPTER 9: RENEWING VOCATIONAL CREATIVITY

[1]Donald L. Nathanson, *Shame and Pride: Affect, Sex, and the Birth of Self* (New York: W. W. Norton, 1992), pp. 326, 360.

[2]C. S. Lewis, *The Last Battle* (New York: HarperCollins, 1956), pp. 198-203.

[3]N. T. Wright, *Surprised by Hope* (New York: HarperCollins, 2008), p. 46.

[4]David Schrader, personal communication with the author, spring 2012. Dave is a partner with the Full Circle Group, a global consultancy focused on leadership and business development and performance.

# Bibliography

Benner, David. *The Gift of Being Yourself.* Downers Grove, IL: InterVarsity Press, 2004.

Brown, Brené. *Daring Greatly.* New York: Gotham, 2012.

Cozolino, Louis. *The Neuroscience of Human Relationships.* New York: W. W. Norton, 2006.

Dweck, Carol. *Mindset: The Psychology of Success.* New York: Ballantine, 2006.

Eccleston, Alex, Natalie DeWitt, Chris Gunter, Barbara Marte and Deepa Nath. "Epigenetics." *Nature Insight* 447, no. 7143 (2007).

Fosha, Diana, Daniel J. Siegel and Marion F. Solomon. *The Healing Power of Emotion.* New York: W. W. Norton, 2009.

Gottman, John. *The Seven Principles for Making Marriage Work.* New York: Three Rivers Press, 1999.

Karlin, Daniel. *Robert Browning: Selected Poems.* New York: Penguin, 1989.

Langer, Ellen. *The Power of Mindful Learning.* New York: Perseus, 1997.

Lewis, C. S. *A Grief Observed.* New York: Bantam Books, 1976.

———. *The Last Battle.* New York: HarperCollins, 1956.

———. *The Weight of Glory.* New York: HarperCollins, 1949.

Lewis, Michael. *Shame: The Exposed Self.* New York: Simon & Schuster, 1992.

Nathanson, Donald L. *Shame and Pride: Affect, Sex, and the Birth of Self.* New York: W. W. Norton, 1992.

———. Interview by David Boulton. *Children of the Code.* September 8, 2003. www.childrenofthecode.org/interviews/nathanson.htm.

Newbigin, Lesslie. *The Gospel in a Pluralist Society.* Grand Rapids: Eerdmans, 1989.

Polanyi, Michael. *Personal Knowledge.* Chicago: University of Chicago Press, 1958.

Schore, Allan. *Affect Regulation and the Repair of the Self.* New York: W. W. Norton, 2003.

Serkin, Peter. *Divine and Human.* Grand Rapids: Zondervan, 2000.

Siegel, Daniel J. *The Developing Mind.* New York: Guilford, 1999.

———. *The Mindful Brain.* New York: W. W. Norton, 2007.

———. *Mindsight.* New York: Bantam, 2010.

———. *The Neurobiology of We: How Relationships, the Mind, and the Brain Interact to Shape Who We Are.* Louisville, CO: Sounds True Audio, 2008.

Siegel, Daniel J., and Mary Hartzell. *Parenting from the Inside Out.* New York: Penguin, 2003.

Thompson, Curt. *Anatomy of the Soul.* Carol Stream, IL: Tyndale House, 2010.

Tomkins, Silvan. *Affect Imagery Consciousness: The Complete Edition.* New York: Springer, 2008.

Wilder, E. James, Edward Khouri, Chris Coursey and Sheila D. Sutton. *Joy Starts Here.* East Peoria, IL: Shepherd's House, 2013.

Wilson, Timothy. *Strangers to Ourselves.* Cambridge, MA: Harvard University Press, 2002.

Wright, N. T. *Surprised by Hope.* New York: HarperCollins, 2008.